essential homeopathy

Books by Dana Ullman

essential homeopathy

what it is & what it can do for you

DANA ULLMAN, M.P.H.

New World Library
Novato, California
www.newworldlibrary.com

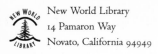

New World Library
14 Pamaron Way
Novato, California 94949

Library of Congress Cataloging-in-Publication Data
Ullman, Dana.
 Essential homeopathy : what it is and what it can do for you
 / Dana Ullman.
     p.   cm.
Includes bibliographical references and index.
 ISBN 1-57731-206-6
 I. Homeopathy—Popular works. I. Title.
 RX76 .U4535 2002
 615.5′32—dc21   2001005837

First Printing, January 2002
ISBN: 1-57731-206-6
Printed in Canada on acid-free, recycled paper
Distributed to the trade by Publishers Group West

10 9 8 7 6 5 4 3 2 1

CONTENTS

introduction

Homeopathy has been called the grandfather of alternative medicine in the United States because it was the first popular medical treatment practiced by medical doctors as a distinct alternative to conventional therapies of the nineteenth century. However, soon after the turn of the twentieth century, aggressive attacks by the American Medical Association (A.M.A.) led to its decline in the United States. Despite this decline in the States, homeopathy maintained its popularity throughout the world, and it is now so popular in Europe that in many countries it is no longer appropriate to consider it "alternative medicine."

And although homeopathy is still not completely

understood or respected in the United States, this attitude is changing rapidly. A growing body of research is verifying homeopathy's efficacy. An increasing number of health and medical professionals are integrating it into their medical practice, and a renaissance of interest among consumers is bringing further attention to it.

Even America's most respected doctor, Dr. C. Everett Koop, has acknowledged in his autobiography that it was his experience as a child with his family doctor, a homeopathic physician, that inspired him to become a doctor. England's most well-known advocate of homeopathy is the queen herself. In fact, the royal family has sought homeopathic care since the 1830s, making homeopathy almost as much a part of the royal tradition as the passing of the crown.

But homeopathy is not just for royalty. It is used by physicians and consumers all over the world to treat common minor ailments, infectious diseases, injuries, chronic diseases, mental illness, and even some genetic ailments. Homeopathic medicines cannot cure everything, of course, but as you read this book, you will be surprised and even amazed at what you learn about the power of homeopathic medicines not only to provide relief but also to promote real and profound healing.

using this book

Whether you are new to homeopathy or are knowledgeable and experienced in the field, this book will provide a clear and precise overview of this magnificent system of natural medicine.

Many people commonly mistake and misconstrue homeopathic medicines as some type of folk medicines or herbal remedies. Chapter 1 clarifies what homeopathy is (and what it isn't). Chapter 2 describes what types of medicinal substances are used in homeopathy and how these substances are made into homeopathic remedies. The fact that homeopathic medicines are made into such infinitesimal doses is counterintuitive to most rational people. Yet homeopathy has been used for more than two hundred years by hundreds of thousands of doctors all over the world. Further, a large body of high-quality scientific studies has been published in respected medical journals that verify the biological activity and clinical efficacy of homeopathic medicine. Chapter 3 reviews this scientific evidence.

If homeopathic medicines are so effective, then why isn't homeopathy more popular? You will probably be amazed to learn that homeopathy is extremely popular in many countries in Europe, Asia, and South America. Although homeopathy isn't presently very popular in the United States, there are specific political and economic reasons for this. The attack against homeopathy by the American Medical Association is one reason for homeopathy's diminished status, and the details of this drama are discussed in chapter 4.

While one can learn to treat oneself and one's family with homeopathic medicines for many common acute ailments, it is necessary to seek out professional homeopathic care for any serious or chronic ailments. Chapter 5 describes who homeopaths are, what training they receive, how to choose one, and whether insurance covers their care. Chapter 6 and 7 highlight some of the remedies that you can use to treat common ailments. Remember: People who take their disease lying down are apt to stay that way. *You* are the most important member of your health-care team, and you can easily learn to use some simple homeopathic medicines to treat yourself and your family. Finally, the "Homeopathy Resources" section at the back of the book is invaluable. A book like this can only plant a seed and introduce you to basic information about the science and art of homeopathy. I strongly encourage you to access other books, tapes, software, and organizations so that you can get the most from this amazingly effective system of healing.

CHAPTER 1

what is homeopathy?

Most people have had some experience with homeopathy, from noticing remedies at the health food store to trying them out themselves to seeing a professional homeopath. But many have only a vague idea of what homeopathic medicine really is. In this chapter I will provide a brief explanation of homeopathy and how it works.

Homeopathic medicine is a natural pharmaceutical science that uses various plants, minerals, or animal products in very small doses to stimulate the sick person's natural defenses. In Greek the word *homoios* means "similar," and *pathos* means "disease" or "suffering." The basic principle of homeopathy is called the "law of similars," because medicines are individually chosen for their ability to cause in overdose in healthy people the symptoms similar to what the sick person experiences.

In essence, homeopathy consists of two highly systematic methods: toxicology and case taking. First, homeopaths discern the specific physical, emotional, and mental symptoms that various substances cause in overdose. In fact, homeopathic texts contain more details about toxicology than any other sources. Second, homeopaths interview their patients in great detail to learn about all the symptoms — physical, emotional, and mental — the patient is experiencing. The homeopath ultimately seeks to find a substance that will cause symptoms similar to what the person experiences and then gives it in small, specially prepared doses.

the principle of similars

Homeopaths, like many modern physiologists, recognize that symptoms represent the best efforts of the organism to adapt to and defend against various stresses or infections. Because the body is not always successful in dealing with every stress or infection on its own, it is important to find substances in nature with the capacity to aid the body in its efforts to defend and ultimately heal itself. Thus the medicines go *with*, rather than *against*, the person's natural defenses.

The principle of similars, the primary premise of homeopathy, is even used in some conventional medical therapies, such as immunizations and allergy treatments. These treatments, however, are not pure homeopathy, since homeopathic medicines are more individually pre-scribed, given in smaller doses, and used to treat sick people *and* to prevent disease. Ultimately, homeopaths, and more traditional doctors, prescribe according to the "principle of similars" because it works.

our inner doctor

Homeopathy, like conventional physiology and pathol-ogy, recognizes that symptoms do not simply represent something "wrong" with the person but rather that they are actually the body's defense against infection and/or stress. The body creates symptoms in its effort to defend and heal itself.

Every textbook on pathology recognizes that inflam-mation is the body's way to heat up, burn out, and isolate infective organisms. Although conventional anti-inflammatory drugs work temporarily to reduce inflam-mation, they do not influence the underlying cause of the inflammation. Such drugs provide a short-term benefit but often lead to longer-term complications.

The human organism has survived as long as it has because we have an "inner doctor" who helps us fight infection and adapt to stress. Using conventional drugs to inhibit or suppress symptoms tends to push the dis-ease deeper into our bodies, creating more serious chronic physical and mental illness. The homeopathic principle of similars, on the other hand, respects the body's own wisdom and seeks to find the correct, individualized remedy that will mimic and augment this wisdom.

how do you know when you're cured?

Although many people believe that they are cured when either a conventional or natural remedy erases their symptoms, that's not necessarily true. Just because a person's symptoms disappear doesn't mean that she is better off, and in fact, it may mean that she is in fact sicker.

For instance, we commonly recognize that people who suppress emotions tend to explode later, usually to some unsuspecting soul. Likewise, many conventional drugs work by inhibiting or actually suppressing the disease, which ultimately pushes the disease deeper into the person, creating more serious and often chronic illnesses that manifest later. This is called "disease suppression." What are often called the "side effects" of a drug are usually the results of this suppression.

Between cure and disease suppression is "palliation," that is, a treatment that provides temporary relief of an illness but does not suppress it. Palliative treatments are given when the person's immune system is reasonably strong. Although the treatment used does not cure the disease, it does provide enough relief to the person that his body is able to avoid disease suppression.

To evaluate whether a cure, palliation, or suppression

has occurred, it is useful first to understand Hering's guidelines to cure.

hering's guidelines to cure

Constantine Hering, M.D. (1800–1880), is considered the father of American homeopathy. He observed that patients often get better in somewhat predictable patterns. Hering recognized that each person experiences a specific pattern of symptoms, and that when comparing this pattern with past or future ones, it is necessary to evaluate the degree to which the symptoms cause pain and discomfort and the degree to which they inhibit a person's life. Hering assumed, for example, that skin symptoms are superficial signs of deeper, internal physical symptoms, that mild irritability is considerably less limiting than a fear of death, and that minor memory problems are significantly less problematic than, say, schizophrenia.

Hering and others since him have developed ways to evaluate the depth and breadth of physical, emotional, and mental/spiritual levels of a person's health. He and other homeopaths have found that certain symptoms in each level of a person's health, depending on their frequency and intensity, represent more and more serious stresses to that person's health.

Based on these assumptions, Hering developed guidelines to help us understand how to differentiate a healing response from a disruptive or diseasing response.

His guidelines to cure were based on the premise that a curative response evolves:

1. from the most vital functions of the person to more superficial ones (a healing process will indicate that a person with a high fever or high blood pressure will experience a reduction in fever or blood pressure, while other less vital physical symptoms may increase as a way of helping to externalize the disease process);
2. from internal sources to external ones (sometimes mental or emotional symptoms will decrease, while more superficial physical symptoms may increase); and
3. in reverse order of appearance (a person may re-experience symptoms that were either previously suppressed or never fully cured as a way to finally get rid of them).

These insights are useful no matter what treatment, conventional or natural, one uses.

discerning what works

Homeopathy is actually based on thousands of experiments in which human subjects have taken continual doses of various plant, mineral, or animal substances until specific symptoms were elicited. These experiments are called "provings," and they are conducted on humans, not animals, because homeopaths believe that the symptoms a substance causes in an animal do not necessarily accurately parallel how the substance will act on the human body.

Innumerable substances cause skin rashes, digestive problems, tumors, and various other disease processes; however, each substance causes its own unique pattern of symptoms. The trick to making a homeopathic medicine work is finding the medicine that matches the overall pattern of symptoms that the person is experiencing, not just a single symptom or small group of symptoms.

Once it is known what a substance causes in overdose, the specific affinity that this substance has to the human body is then understood. And because symptoms represent the best defense of the human body to fight infection and/or to adapt to stress, it makes sense to mimic and augment the body's own defenses.

the importance of individualized medicine

In homeopathy you don't simply treat the disease; you treat the person, who will have his own manifestation of a disease, as well as many other symptoms that are a part of his unique ailment. Therefore, it is essential to individualize a homeopathic treatment to the person receiving it.

A person does not simply have a heart problem when he has heart disease, and a person does not simply have a skin problem when she has skin disease. Disease is rarely localized to one part of the person. The whole person is ill, not just an isolated part. Ultimately, a person's illness is an overall syndrome, of which the disease is but a part.

For instance, people with arthritis (or with any disease) generally have many symptoms in common, but each person also has many symptoms that are unique to him or her. Based on this important point of view, it is scientifically unsound to treat everyone with a similar disease with the same drug.

treat the person, not the disease

Two people may have a headache, but each will have his or her own pattern of symptoms or syndrome. It is remarkable how misinformed we have been in thinking that everyone with a headache has the same condition and should be treated similarly.

A person suffering from a headache may also have digestive complaints, respiratory problems, skin symptoms, psychological problems, and many other possible symptoms. Because each person is an individual, it is inappropriate (and ineffective) to treat each complaint that a person experiences as a separate condition. In homeopathy, one seeks to find an individualized remedy that fits the person's overall pattern or syndrome of symptoms.

William Osler, M.D., considered the father of modern medicine, once said, "It is more important to know what type of person has a disease than what type of disease a person has." This is the assumption behind homeopathic medicine.

CHAPTER 2

how homeopathic medicines are made

In this chapter I will describe how homeopathic medicines are made, including a discussion of what ingredients are used and why these substances are such potent healing agents. I will also discuss prescriptions and dosages of these medicines.

types of medicines used in homeopathy

Various substances from the plant, mineral, or animal kingdoms are regularly used in homeopathy, and almost any type of material can become a homeopathic medicine. Once a homeopathic "proving" is conducted (an experiment done to discover what a substance causes in overdose and thus what it will cure in homeopathic dose), it is then known how that medicine can be useful when given in homeopathic doses.

Some homeopathic medicines from the plant kingdom include onion *(Allium cepa)*, ipecac root *(Ipecacuahna)*, and poison ivy *(Rhus toxicodendron)*. Some homeopathic medicines from the mineral kingdom include calcium *(Calcarea carbonate)*, arsenic *(Arsenicum)*, and salt *(Natrum muriaticum)*. Some homeopathic medicines from the animal kingdom include bee venom *(Apis mellifica)*, rattlesnake venom *(Crotalus horridus)*, and dog's milk *(Lac caninum)*. It should be noted that homeopathic medicines are listed by their Latin name, because homeopaths insist on being precise in describing the specific species they use in their medicines.

You might be asking why substances such as snake venom and arsenic are used in homeopathic remedies. Various strange and even poisonous substances are used in homeopathy because they have been found to cause a pattern of symptoms similar to what sick people experience. Therefore, by taking small, specially prepared doses of these substances, one can eliminate their toxic effects while maintaining their healing benefits. Homeopaths use such small doses of these substances that even homeopathy's strongest critics assert that homeopathic medicines are basically safe.

It should also be noted that although homeopathy uses strange substances, so does every system of medicine. Conventional medicine uses drugs derived from mold (penicillin) and pregnant horse's urine (Premarin), to list but a few examples, yet few people call physicians "witch doctors" for doing so.

some examples of homeopathic medicines

When you are chopping an onion, your eyes tear up, and you might experience a watery, burning discharge from your nose. These symptoms are aggravated when you are in a warm room, and they are reduced if the room is cool. Homeopathic doses of onion *(Allium cepa)* are used to treat people with a cold or allergies if they exhibit similar symptoms. If, however, a person with a cold has a stringy yellow nasal discharge that is aggravated by exposure to cold or open air, then a medicine using onion is not prescribed but rather *Kali bichromicum* (potassium bichromate).

It is initially confusing but ultimately logical that homeopaths use ipecac root *(Ipecacuanha)* to treat people with certain types of nausea and vomiting. It is commonly known that ipecac root causes nausea and vomiting, and because of this, it has an important place in emergency medicine as a method of inducing vomiting if someone has ingested certain poisons. In homeopathy, *Ipecacuanha* is used to treat people who experience symptoms similar to what *Ipecacuanha* is known to cause: constant nausea with no relief from vomiting, lack of thirst with increased salivation, and a clean pinkish tongue despite indigestion.

how homeopathic medicines are made

Homeopathic medicines are made through a specific pharmaceutical process called "potentization." With plant or liquid substances, the tincture of the plant is extracted, usually through distillation with alcohol. The solution is then diluted with one part of the tincture with nine or ninety-nine parts of a double-distilled purified water. This new solution is vigorously shaken (or "succussed"), and then the dilution and succussion process is repeated numerous times. Typically, a homeopathic medicine is potentized three, six, twelve, thirty, two hundred, one thousand, ten thousand, fifty thousand, one hundred thousand times, or more. When mineral substances are used, they are triturated (ground up) with lactose (milk sugar). Initially, one part of the mineral substance is ground together with nine or ninety-nine parts of lactose. Each substance is diluted and then triturated up to thirty times, and then it is dissolved into a double-distilled water, at which time it is potentized in a process similar to that used with plant or liquid substances.

single- and multiple-ingredient medicines

"Single-ingredient" homeopathic medicines use various plant, mineral, animal, or chemical substances that have undergone a proving. Classical homeopathy uses single-ingredient remedies and has been practiced for more than two hundred years. However, many homeopathic manufacturers create formulas that are combinations of various homeopathic ingredients. Generally, a manufacturer creates a formula by combining two to ten of the most common remedies used to treat a specific ailment (headache, allergies, arthritis, and so on). Although these formulas are not individually prescribed, they are often effective at least in providing temporary relief, and they are considerably safer than most conventional drugs, because homeopathic remedies are nontoxic.

Some classical homeopaths assert that these formulas are not "real homeopathy," since the medicines have not undergone their own provings and because they are not individualized to the person. While these critiques are certainly true, the ingredients are homeopathically prepared and, more important, they have been found to work reasonably well.

In general, individually chosen remedies tend to work better; however, it should be acknowledged that such individually chosen remedies only work better if the person prescribing them was adequately educated in finding the correct remedy. Most laypeople are not trained in homeopathy, so homeopathic formulas provide a "user-friendly" way for people to use these natural medicines.

over-the-counter remedies

In the United States, homeopathic medicines are legally recognized as "over-the-counter drugs"; that is, they do not require a prescription from a medical doctor. All over-the-counter drugs, including homeopathic remedies, are required by the Federal Drug Administration (F.D.A.) to provide a disease indication for conditions that do not require a medical diagnosis or ongoing medical monitoring and that are self-limiting (that is, they are not fatal and will resolve themselves at some point). Colds, influenza, sore throat, allergies, sinusitis, P.M.S., teething, colic, headaches, and arthritis are but some examples of these conditions. If you see homeopathic medicines marketed for heart disease, diabetes, cancer, multiple sclerosis, or any serious or fatal illness, you are encouraged to contact the F.D.A. in Washington, D.C.

how safe are homeopathic medicines?

The small doses used in homeopathic medicines make these medicines extremely safe. Of course, it is important to know how to prescribe the medicines. The book I co-authored with Dr. Stephen Cummings, *Everybody's Guide to Homeopathic Medicines,* provides step-by-step information on how to use the medicines and when it is necessary to seek medical care.

Within a given year, it is common for the F.D.A. to not receive a single report of any problems or complications resulting from a homeopathic medicine. And because they are recognized as drugs, their manufacture is regulated by the F.D.A. to assure consumers that they are getting what they ordered.

the scientific evidence

Homeopathy is gaining increasing international attention, and this attention is in part the result of a growing body of research supporting the positive results that people commonly experience. Yet homeopathy is still widely misunderstood. In this chapter I hope to clear up some of the more common misconceptions about homeopathy.

Many people believe, for example, that because homeopathic doses are so small they couldn't possibly work. Actually, there are many examples from nature of extremely small doses having powerful effects. Pheromones, for example, are hormones that are emitted from the bodies of many animals — including human beings — and that let them seek out and tell others of their own species that they wish to mate. Certain species of moths can smell another of their own species even if they are two miles away. Further, there are innumerable examples of various animals' ability to smell or sense extremely low concentrations of certain things necessary for their survival. Sharks, for instance, can smell blood in the ocean, which helps them to find food, even at great distances. When one considers the volume of water in the ocean, it seems obvious that the sharks are sensing extremely small amounts of blood.

There are also numerous examples involving human beings. Some people who are allergic to cats, for instance, can develop strong symptoms even if only one cat walked through a room several hours or days earlier.

clinical evidence

The results of some very good scientific research have been published in medical journals and other scientific publications. The *Lancet* published a review of eighty-nine double-blind or randomized placebo-controlled clinical trials (Linde et al. 1997) in which the authors conclude that the clinical effects of homeopathic medicines are unlikely to be simply the results of a placebo effect. In fact, they found that homeopathic medicines had a 2.45 times greater effect than placebos did. The lead author of this review of homeopathic research, Klaus Linde, M.D., was the same German professor who reviewed the research on St. John's wort that received international attention.

Another survey of research published in the *British Medical Journal* indicated that 81 out of 107 controlled clinical trials showed that homeopathic medicines had beneficial results (Kleijnen et al. 1991). For more details about many of these studies, see my book *The Consumer's Guide to Homeopathy* or *The Emerging Science of Homeopathy* (Bellavite and Signorini 2002).

homeopathic microdoses do work

The advantage of most good laboratory studies on homeopathy is that even skeptics cannot propose that the effects are placebo effects. This type of research does not try to verify clinical efficacy; instead, it simply seeks to verify if the small doses used in homeopathy cause any type of biological effect. In fact, there are dozens of such studies. This book simply highlights a few.

One recent study that was replicated by four research institutes in Europe found that homeopathic doses of histamine had a dramatic effect on one type of white blood cell (Belon et al. 1999). In particular, the researchers found that the 15C to 19C potencies of histamine had significant effects.

A French hematologist has repeatedly found that homeopathic doses of aspirin have significant effects on reducing bleeding time and on platelet aggregation and coagulation (Belougne-Malfatti et al. 1998). Because aspirin in normal or high doses increases bleeding time, it was predicted that homeopathic doses would reduce it, and this study verified this prediction.

A highly respected German professor and a group of researchers conducted a meta-analysis of 105 studies in which researchers used homeopathic doses of various heavy metals or other toxic substances as a way to prevent disease or death in animals that were exposed to overdoses of these same toxic substances (Linde, Jonas, Melchart et al. 1994). When reviewing just the well-done studies, the researchers found a consistent pattern of efficacy from the homeopathic doses, which, on average, helped the animal excrete approximately 20 percent more of the toxic substance through its urine, stools, or sweat.

One of the researchers in this mostly German team was Wayne Jonas, an American medical doctor who was also a lieutenant colonel in the United States Army. He and other researchers at the Walter Reed Army Institute investigated the protective effects of homeopathic doses of glutamate on different types of rat cells. Glutamate is an amino acid that is an important nutrient in small doses but is toxic in highly concentrated doses (Jonas, Lin, and Tortella 2001). The researchers found significant protective effects of homeopathic doses of glutamate, including at doses that conventional scientific wisdom suggests are so small that there should be no remaining molecules of glutamate in the medicinal solution.

more evidence

Homeopathy became popular in this country and in Europe during the 1800s because of its success in treating the many infectious diseases that raged then, including yellow fever, scarlet fever, and cholera. The death rate in homeopathic hospitals was between one-half to one-eighth of that in conventional medical hospitals. It is hard to imagine that these significant results in treating serious infectious disease were due to a placebo effect.

Homeopathic medicines also have been shown to work on infants and on various animals (including dogs, cats, horses, and cows), creatures seemingly incapable of experiencing the placebo effect. Homeopaths also find that people who are being treated with homeopathic medicine for a chronic disease sometimes experience a temporary exacerbation in their symptoms as the body's defenses are being stimulated. Homeopaths have found that a "healing crisis" is sometimes necessary to achieve healing. It is highly unlikely that this temporary worsening of symptoms is the result of a placebo response.

Remember that the small doses used by homeopaths only have an effect when the person taking the remedy has a hypersensitivity to the small doses given. If the wrong medicine is given to a person, nothing happens. If the correct medicine is given, it acts as a catalyst to the person's defenses. In any case, homeopathic medicines do not have side effects.

how homeopathic medicines work

Despite the vast amount of research conducted on conventional drugs today sponsored by large drug companies or by the federal government, there are many commonly used drugs that we still don't understand. Likewise, we do not know precisely how homeopathic medicines work.

Research has found that the water in which homeopathic medicines are made emits more heat, which might contribute to the medicines' effect. A former professor of physics at the California Institute of Technology has found that once a double-distilled purified water is sequentially diluted and shaken with a medicinal substance inside it, an ice crystal that doesn't melt in room-temperature water and that maintains an electrical field is created (Lo and Bonavida 1997; Gray 2000). Dr. Lo has even taken electron microscope photos of these crystals. How these crystals work on the body, however, remains a mystery.

There are various other theories about how homeopathic medicines work, some of which are highly technical (see Bellavite and Signorini 2002). Some people assume that the highly potentized homeopathic medicines are "energy medicines" that act on the *chi*, or "life energy" of the person. It is then assumed that the more potentized the medicine, the more energetic it is, and the deeper it acts on the person's energy.

It should also be noted that submarines communicate

with other submarines and with ships using very low radio frequencies, because higher frequencies cannot penetrate the water. Because the human being is 75 to 80 percent water, very low doses of medicines, such as those used in homeopathic medicine, may be a more effective means of delivering drugs than the high doses commonly used in conventional medicine.

One of the hottest subjects in science today is "nanotechnologies." *Nano* is a prefix referring to the study and use of hyperminiaturized technologies that can carry more and more bodies of information in smaller and smaller chips. In this spirit, it may be appropriate to refer to homeopathy as a "nanopharmacology."

a brief history
of homeopathy

The founder of homeopathic medicine was Samuel Hahnemann, M.D. (1755–1843), a German physician and chemist. Although Hahnemann developed the system of homeopathy, its principles are ancient and have been used in many cultures. Hippocrates wrote about and used the principle of similars, and the Mayans and the Incas used them.

Hahnemann quit his own medical practice because he felt that he was doing more harm than good (historians today recognize that physicians of Hahnemann's day did indeed do more harm than good). He was a scholar, and he was able to make a living translating books. And because he was a sophisticated experimenter, he sought to prove or disprove the ancient principle of similars. He did this by conducting provings, experimenting first on himself, then on his family, and then on his students. These provings only used human subjects and sought to discover what symptoms various substances from the plant, mineral, and animal kingdoms caused in overdose. Once it was known what they caused in overdose, Hahnemann and others then learned what they could potentially heal when prescribed in extremely small, specially prepared doses.

the growth of homeopathy

Homeopathy grew rapidly in Europe and in the United States in the nineteenth century, in part because conventional medicine was so dangerous and in part because homeopathic practitioners and patients were obtaining impressive results in treating the many infectious disease epidemics that raged at that time. The first homeopath came to America in 1825, and it spread so rapidly that by 1844 the American Institute of Homeopathy was formed. Although homeopathic doctors were considerably smaller in number than were conventional doctors, they were the first to form a national medical organization in the United States. Two years later, another medical organization was formed, and they stated in their charter that one of its missions was to stop the growth of homeopathy. That organization called itself the American Medical Association.

Shortly after the formation of the A.M.A., this conventional medical organization forbade their members from talking or consulting with homeopathic doctors or homeopathic patients. Even when William Seward, the secretary of state, was stabbed on the same night that President Lincoln was shot, the surgeon general was reprimanded for providing care to Seward simply because Seward's regular physician was a homeopath. This antagonism against homeopathy was much more the result of emotional and economic issues than of scientific disagreement.

In a 1903 meeting of the A.M.A., a Kentucky physician asserted, "We must admit that we have never fought the homeopath on matters of principles; we fought him because he came into the community and got the business." Homeopathy posed an additional threat because it represented a new and safer way to heal people. A book that won the Pultizer Prize in 1982 noted, "Because homeopathy was simultaneously philosophical and experimental, it seemed to many people to be more rather than less scientific than orthodox medicine." (Starr 1982)

And distinct from other natural therapies that were gaining popularity in the nineteenth century, such as chiropractic, naturopathy, herbology, and osteopathy, the vast majority of homeopaths were medical doctors.

At homeopathy's height in the late nineteenth century, there were twenty-two homeopathic medical schools, including Boston University, the University of Michigan, New York Medical College, Hahnemann

University, the University of Minnesota, and the University of Iowa. There were also more than one hundred homeopathic hospitals and approximately one thousand pharmacies that sold homeopathic medicines. Even many of this country's educated elite were advocates of homeopathy, including Mark Twain, William James, Henry Wadsworth Longfellow, Henry David Thoreau, Nathaniel Hawthorne, Harriet Beecher Stowe, and Louisa May Alcott, among many others.

homeopathy's present status

Homeopathy is still quite popular today throughout the world. It is particularly popular in France, England, Germany, Greece, India, Pakistan, Brazil, Argentina, Mexico, and South Africa. Approximately 40 percent of the French public have used homeopathic medicines, and between 30 and 40 percent of French physicians have prescribed homeopathic medicines. About 20 percent of German physicians occasionally use these natural medicines, and 45 percent of Dutch physicians consider them effective. According to a survey in the *British Medical Journal*, 42 percent of British physicians surveyed refer patients to homeopathic physicians. Homeopathy is particularly popular in India, where there are more than one hundred twenty five-year homeopathic medical schools.

Homeopathy is also growing very rapidly in the United States. Market research shows that sales of homeopathic medicines have grown at a rate of 5 to 20 percent per year during the past ten years, and similar rates of impressive growth are expected in the years to come.

As a sign of homeopathy's growing popularity, according to various reports in the media, the following are but a handful of famous people who use or who have used homeopathic medicines: Lindsay Wagner, Tina Turner, Jane Fonda, Jane Seymour, Whoopi Goldberg, Rosie O'Donnell, Angelica Houston, Muriel Hemingway, Sissy Spacek, Paul McCartney, Priscilla Presley, Linda Gray, Martin Sheen, Nick Nolte, Julianna Margulies, Olivia Newton-John, Michael Franks, Cybil Sheppard, Ashley Judd, Naomi Judd, Vidal Sassoon, Lesley Anne Warren, Axel Rose, Marlene Dietrich, Michael York, Courtney Thorne-Smith, Jackson Pollock, Jerry Hall, Nancy Sinatra, and Cher.

Various media sources have also reported on numerous leading sports figures who have used or still use homeopathic medicines, including Miami Heat coach Pat Riley, New York Yankee Paul O'Neill, tennis star Boris Becker, Olympian Greg Louganis, Jose Maria Olazabal (twice winner of the Masters Golf Tournament), Giants player Jeff Kent, English rugby player Will Greenwood, former Yankee pitcher Jim Bouton, and pro golfer Sally Little.

homeopathy's legal status in the united states

I've had many people ask me if homeopathy is legal in this country. The answer is, Certainly! Most of its practitioners are conventionally trained medical doctors who have furthered their training with the study of homeopathy. Some of its practitioners are other types of health professionals, including dentists, podiatrists, psychologists, physician's assistants, nurses, naturopaths, chiropractors, and even veterinarians.

Some laypeople have also seriously studied homeopathy and are very good practitioners, though the legal issues surrounding their practice remain unclear. Because homeopathic medicines are legally considered "drugs," some authorities assume that anyone who prescribes or recommends them needs to be a physician or have a license to prescribe drugs. However, because the vast majority of homeopathic medicines are considered over-the-counter, which means that consumers do not need a prescription to purchase them, some authorities assume that one does not need a license to use them. Homeopathic practice by unlicensed individuals may be legal if done under the supervision of a physician, but this physician would assume all legal responsibilities for patient care.

The history of homeopathy has only been briefly reviewed here. People who are interested in the conflicts between the homeopaths and the orthodox physicians are encouraged to read my book *Discovering Homeopathy* and Dr. Harris Coulter's *Divided Legacy: The Conflict Between Homeopathy and the American Medical Association.* We can only hope that we learn to get beyond the drama and the conflict between the various schools of medical thought and practice to create an integrated health-care system.

professional
homeopathic care

Deciding when it is appropriate to self-prescribe and when to consult a professional homeopath can be a confusing process. In this chapter, I will describe when professional homeopathic care is strongly indicated, as well as the ins and outs of professional homeopathic care, including what conditions most warrant this type of care, the costs involved in seeking professional treatment, and what to look for in a homeopath.

In general, any recurrent, chronic, severe, or potentially life-threatening conditions require professional homeopathic attention. That said, homeopaths usually encourage self-care for common acute, non-life-threatening ailments and injuries. The majority of symptoms that people commonly experience stem from conditions that they can treat (and heal) themselves. People can also treat themselves for many relatively mild chronic ailments, such as allergies, headaches, sinusitis, arthritic pain, and P.M.S. However, such self-care at best provides temporary relief, while professional homeopathic care provides the potential for a real significant improvement, even a cure.

The special services that professional homeopaths provide include prescribing a "constitutional remedy," that is, a remedy individually prescribed based on your genetic heritage, your health history, your body type, your psychological type, and the totality of physical and psychological symptoms that you are presently experiencing. A constitutional remedy has the potential to provide a profound strengthening of your general well-being.

Because the correct homeopathic constitutional medicines can so deeply improve a person's overall state of health, professional homeopathic care makes sense for almost any person at least at some time in his or her life. There are, in particular, eight primary indications for seeking professional homeopathic care:

1. Disease prevention and health promotion
2. Genetic disorders
3. Prepregnancy and pregnancy
4. Recurrent subtle symptoms
5. Serious acute symptoms
6. Recurrent injuries

7. Chronic ailments

8. Debilitating or recurrent psychological problems

Despite the great potential of homeopathic constitutional remedies, please keep in mind that such remedies are not cure-alls. Depending on a person's health history, these remedies can sometimes be limited in their effectiveness.

disease prevention and health promotion

The professional homeopath's prescription of a constitutional medicine for each patient has the potential for preventing many diseases, diminishing the potential impact from many ailments, and creating an overall higher level of health. Even if a person is relatively healthy, he or she can benefit from these treatments.

genetic disorders

Homeopathy cannot usually cure genetic diseases, but it can strengthen a person against their effects. For instance, the homeopathic treatment of a child with Down's syndrome will not cure this genetic condition, but the child will not experience as many infections as other children with Down's syndrome and will tend to achieve a higher degree of intelligence.

A person with diabetes who undergoes homeopathic care will still have diabetes, but he or she may not require as much insulin, may not need to maintain as strict a diet, and may not experience as many complications from the disease as diabetics not under homeopathic care.

People with genetic diseases tend to require a series of remedies over time to slowly remove the varying layers of disease. Homeopathic medicines cannot do the "impossible," but they commonly surprise both practitioners and patients with powerful healing responses that grant greater health.

prepregnancy and pregnancy

It is always a good idea to see a homeopath during prepregnancy and pregnancy, for several reasons. First, homeopaths have clinically found that homeopathic medicines create better overall health in people, thereby increasing the chances of becoming pregnant and of completing the pregnancy. Second, homeopaths have long observed that pregnant women respond particularly well to homeopathic medicines, and because improved health of the mother tends to lead to better health of the fetus, it makes sense to consider using homeopathic remedies during pregnancy. Whether the woman experiences common symptoms of pregnancy such as nausea, fatigue, and hemorrhoids or has her own unique symptoms, homeopathic remedies can provide effective and safe relief. Last, physicians today finally recognize the danger of using conventional drugs during pregnancy. All drugs seem to penetrate the placental barrier, and it is not known which will have only minor effects and which will create serious health problems. Homeopathic medicines provide a considerably safer alternative.

In addition, women who are breastfeeding will benefit from professional homeopathic care, as will their babies.

recurrent subtle symptoms

It is quite common for relatively healthy people to suffer from minor symptoms such as low energy at certain times of the day; hypersensitivity to heat or cold; irregularities in bowel movements, urination, or sweat; sleeping problems; menstrual difficulties; and so on. Many people experience symptoms that are not serious enough for physicians to define the condition in pathological terms yet are serious enough to diminish the person's quality of life.

A professional homeopath does not require a conventional medical diagnosis in order to prescribe an individualized homeopathic medicine that might strengthen the patient and diminish various minor or subtle symptoms that are experienced.

serious acute symptoms

One of the great benefits of homeopathic medicines is that they are often very fast acting, especially when a person's symptoms have a rapid onset and/or are severe. It is also beneficial to know that homeopathic medicines can usually be prescribed concurrently with conventional drugs (although certain conventional drugs, such as corticosteroidal drugs, work by suppressing the immune system, thereby reducing the therapeutic benefits of homeopathic medicines, it is rare for conventional drugs to completely negate the healing effects of homeopathic remedies).

Going to a professional homeopath for the treatment of severe acute symptoms is recommended, because a homeopath is much more likely to find a useful remedy for the sick person than she could do herself.

recurrent injuries

It is easy to learn how to use homeopathic medicines to treat common injuries (see chapter 7). When a person experiences recurrent injuries, there is occasionally some type of bodily weakness that professional homeopathic care can sometimes strengthen.

chronic ailments

Conventional medicine is perhaps at its weakest in the treatment and cure of chronic ailments. At best, conventional medicine manages to suppress, control, and manage the symptoms of people with chronic ailments, though all too often, there are various attendant and often serious side effects that result with this treatment.

In this instance, when conventional medicine is weak, homeopathic medicine is at its best. Because chronic illness results from some type of breakdown in a person's overall health and because homeopathy as a system of healing is primarily orientated toward strengthening a person's overall health, people with chronic illness can greatly benefit from professional homeopathic care.

debilitating or recurrent psychological problems

Homeopathic medicines are effective not only in treating physical illness but also emotional and mental illness. In fact, homeopaths do not make any arbitrary separation between the two kinds of illness. Homeopaths assume that physical illness can create its own psychological symptoms and mental illness can create its own physical ailments. Ultimately, each person is an amalgam of physical and psychological symptoms.

The beauty of the homeopathic method is that homeopaths do not have to know (or guess) which came first, the physical symptoms or the psychological ones. Instead, the homeopath prescribes a medicine to cause body and mind symptoms similar to those the sick person is presently experiencing.

While one can learn to use simple homeopathic remedies to treat common acute psychological problems, professional homeopathic care should be sought for any serious or recurrent emotional or mental problems.

what diseases are homeopaths best at treating?

Homeopaths don't treat "diseases"; they treat people with disease. This isn't just semantics. One person's migraine, arthritis, or allergies are not the same as those of another. It is not the disease that is treated, but the person.

That said, patients tend to get the greatest benefit from professional homeopathic care when they have recurrent or chronic symptoms, but not so serious that significant pathological and structural changes have occurred. It is not that homeopathy has nothing to offer people with more serious ailments; it is just that people with these ailments tend to have more significant immune disorders for which homeopathic care is not as consistently effective.

Homeopathic medicines cannot do the impossible, but well-trained homeopaths often can do the improbable. In other words, although homeopathic medicines cannot cure incurable conditions or certain pathological or structural complaints, they can often provide some relief and some improvement in most people's health.

Further, homeopaths see themselves as a part of a health-care team. Along with receiving homeopathic treatment, patients sometimes need to undergo surgery, and it is sometimes necessary for some people to receive physical therapy (or some other type of body work). Also, nutritional counseling, stress management, and psychological counseling are often useful adjunctive therapies that can help a person's overall health and increase the chances that a homeopathic medicine will act more deeply and for a longer period. Thus, homeopaths can and will refer patients for various types of specialty health care, both within the conventional medical model as well as outside it.

what exactly are homeopaths?

Many people are confused about who and what homeopaths are. This confusion is predictable and understandable, because homeopaths fall into so many different professional categories. The majority of practicing homeopaths are medical doctors, though some are naturopathic doctors, some are chiropractic doctors, some are various other types of health professionals, and some are "professional homeopaths" (that is, unlicensed practitioners who have generally completed at least three years of training and have passed a rigorous examination).

Some practitioners specialize in homeopathy and use its remedies as their primary practice, while others use homeopathy in conjunction with other alternative and conventional therapeutics. Generally, the best homeopaths are those who specialize in homeopathy.

Legal Issues

Anyone can obtain and use homeopathic medicines, because the F.D.A. recognizes them primarily as over-the-counter drugs, and thus, they do not require a doctor's prescription. However, the answer to the question of who can actually engage in the practice of homeopathic medicine is not a simple one.

Because homeopathic medicines are recognized as "drugs" in the United States (even if they are non-prescription drugs), most medical boards assume that one must be a medical doctor or licensed to prescribe over-the-counter drugs. As such, physician's assistants, nurses, and other licensed health professionals can usually prescribe homeopathic medicines under the supervision of a medical doctor. Also, naturopathic doctors who are licensed can prescribe homeopathic medicines. Dentists, podiatrists, and other primary-care professionals can also prescribe them.

In 1976 I was arrested for practicing medicine without a license in Oakland, California. Although I won in an important court settlement, it didn't change a set legal precedent. The court allowed me to continue my health practice under two stipulations:

1. that I do not call myself a medical doctor and that I refer to medical doctors for diagnosis and treatment of any disease;
2. that I sign contracts with my patients that make it clear to them that I treat people, not diseases.

These stipulations made complete sense to me. Although this case didn't change the law, it did provide an example of how one court chose to deal with a complex medical-legal issue.

Training

The study of homeopathic medicine is a lifelong endeavor. Teachers and students of homeopathy readily recognize that attending homeopathic schools is just the beginning of their training.

Most homeopathic schools presently offer three-year programs, usually one weekend per month (some programs offer classes on four consecutive days a month). Classroom lectures are only a small part of the training. The majority of study is done at home with a wide variety of books and assignments. Generally, students are expected to study between one and three hours a day.

Naturopathic medical schools provide some good training in homeopathy. These colleges offer four-year, full-time training programs. The same requirements for getting into conventional medical schools are required for getting into naturopathic schools. A significant amount of clinical instruction is also provided. At present, there are five accredited naturopathic schools in North America (the National College of Naturopathic Medicine in Portland, Oregon; Bastyr University in Seattle, Washington; Southwest College of Naturopathic Medicine in Tempe, Arizona; Bridgeport University in Bridgeport, Connecticut; and Ontario College of Naturopathic Medicine in Toronto, Canada).

There are also some homeopathic correspondence courses. Some of these programs are actually quite good, though as homeopathy grows in popularity, one can expect some programs to be excellent and others to provide inadequate training. Correspondence courses integrate cassette lectures, books, written material, and homework. Some correspondence courses also integrate in-class coursework.

Please note that presently a select group of correspondence schools grant naturopathic degrees (N.D.). These distance-learning programs do not offer any clinical training, and their programs do not approach the depth and breadth of the conventional naturopathic schools listed above. Further, the N.D. degree that one obtains from these correspondence schools does not enable the graduate to apply for or to receive a license to practice naturopathic medicine in any state in the United States. While these programs may provide some useful information on natural healing, the training doesn't match doctoral-level education that most consumers expect from their practitioner.

If you call or visit a naturopath, I recommend that you ask which type of school she or he attended.

types of homeopathy

Some homeopaths use primarily low-potency medicines, and others use primarily high-potency ones. Some recommend a single remedy at a time, while others prescribe several remedies together. Some use only a single dose of a remedy and expect the effects to last from one to twelve months, while others recommend several doses daily for several weeks. And there are variations to each of these approaches. The three most common types of homeopathy are:

- classical homeopathy
- unconventional homeopathy
- formula homeopathy

Classical Homeopathy

"Classical homeopathy" refers to the way in which homeopathy was practiced by its founder, Dr. Samuel Hahnemann, and his closest followers. Classical homeopathy consists of:

- the prescription of a single remedy based on the totality of a person's symptoms;
- the prescription of a remedy based on clinical experience and on experiments called "provings" that delineate the symptoms a substance causes in overdose and cures in microdose;
- using a minimum dose of medicine (because the best homeopathic medicines stimulate a person's body to heal itself, it is not always necessary to repeatedly take doses of a medicine; the best and most effective healing occurs with the minimum number of doses).

Classical homeopaths usually use high-potency medicines (200, 1M, 10M, 50M, and higher; "M" refers to the Roman numeral for one thousand, meaning that they were diluted either 1:10 or 1:100 one thousand times) more than low-potency remedies (3, 6, or 12). Some good homeopaths also use a range of potencies called "LM" potencies, referring to the fact that these are diluted 1:50,000.

Unconventional Homeopathy

"Unconventional homeopathy" is so-called because its methods of prescribing homeopathic medicine are different from those used in classical practice. There are various types of unconventional homeopathy. One style uses numerous (usually two to five) homeopathic medicines concurrently, each of which is individually prescribed for different symptoms a person is experiencing. This method of prescribing multiple homeopathic remedies is commonly practiced in France and Germany.

Practitioners of another type of unconventional homeopathy use various instrumentation or physical tests to find appropriate homeopathic medicines. One type of unconventional homeopathy uses electronic testing devices in which an electrode measures skin conductance at an acupuncture point. Too high or too low skin conductance suggests an imbalance that might be corrected by a homeopathic medicine. To find the correct remedy, practitioners ask the patient to hold on to a homeopathic medicine. The correct remedy will create a balanced reading.

This type of practitioner tends to find individual remedies for each imbalance point, usually leading to the prescription of ten to twenty different remedies. Some practitioners seek to find a smaller number of medicines (usually one to three) that will aid the majority of imbalances. Electronic homeopathy is most commonly practiced in America, Germany, and Italy, though it represents a small group of these countries' homeopaths.

Some practitioners of unconventional homeopathy

use muscle testing, also known as "applied kinesiology." This type of testing measures the strength of specific muscle groupings that are supposedly representative of the person's overall health or of specific systems of the body. Some practitioners use muscle testing to find the correct remedy, while others use this method to assess which potency to use.

One other type of unconventional homeopathy uses hand-held pendulums to help find the correct homeopathic medicines. Pendulums are made from various metals or natural substances that are swung from a metal chain or a string. A homeopathic remedy is placed in the patient's hand, and the pendulum will usually swing clockwise when it is a beneficial medicine for him or her. This method, like most methods of unconventional homeopathy, is quite subjective and tends to be as good as the practitioner's intuition.

An even more mystical method of finding the correct homeopathic medicine is through an instrument called a radionics machine. A description of how radionic machines work may give the impression that they are the epitome of quackery, but actually, an early 1900 version of this technology was developed by the dean of Clinical Medicine at Stanford Medical School, Dr. Albert Abrams. Dr. Abrams would place a sample of a person's blood, sputum, or even a photograph of the individual onto a metal plate in the machine's panel, and then place different medicines near the sample, using a pendulum to determine which medicines are needed. Despite the seemingly quack nature of this device, I have personally witnessed some impressive diagnoses and very impressive treatments with radionics machines.

It may make sense to consult a practitioner of unconventional homeopathy when practitioners of classical homeopathy have not been effective in finding the proper remedies, especially after a year of care. Practitioners of unconventional homeopathy are sometimes able to find rare and unusual remedies that can be extremely effective. They also sometimes uncover unusual genetic tendencies or recent exposure to toxic substances that can be important in selecting the proper homeopathic remedy for the patient.

Although unconventional homeopathy does not usually lead to the discovery of a person's constitutional medicine, these methods sometimes help the practitioner to find a remedy that will enable a constitutional remedy to act powerfully, when the presumably correct constitutional remedy has previously had little or no effect.

The best practitioners of unconventional homeopathy are usually those who know a lot about homeopathy and homeopathic medicines. They do not simply expect their instruments or their testing to provide them with the "answers"; they use their knowledge to find a select number of remedies and then use their modern techniques to distinguish which is the best remedy and its best potency.

Formula Homeopathy

"Formula homeopathy" refers to mixtures in a single bottle of two to ten or so homeopathic medicines that are known to be effective in treating a specific ailment.

Usually, these formulas are marketed for a specific ailment, such as colds, headaches, allergies, arthritis, sinusitis, P.M.S., and sore throats. These formulas are a user-friendly method of taking homeopathic medicine, since they do not require the same high level of individualization used in classical homeopathy.

The logic behind using homeopathic formulas is that at least one of the remedies in the formula may benefit the sick person. It makes sense to use homeopathic formulas when the practitioner doesn't know how to find the individual remedy, when the remedy isn't obvious, or when the individualized remedy isn't immediately available. Formulas may also be indicated at the early stages of an acute ailment when there are few individualizing symptoms. Although homeopathic formulas do not "cure" the patient's chronic disease or underlying ailment, they often provide important temporary relief of a person's complaint.

Most classical practitioners do not usually use homeopathic formulas, relying instead on their professional training to find individualized remedies for sick people. This doesn't mean that the formulas don't work; it simply suggests that the professional homeopath often aspires toward the higher goal of a deep cure, a step beyond temporary relief of symptoms.

how to find a homeopath

The National Center for Homeopathy publishes a directory of homeopaths in the United States and Canada. It is available from them as well as from Homeopathic Educational Services of Berkeley (addresses for these organizations can be found in the resources at the back of this book). In addition to listing homeopathic practitioners, it also lists several hundred homeopathic study groups. These groups of laypeople meet once or twice a month to learn homeopathy together. Homeopathic study groups are usually the best resource for learning about homeopathy and for getting recommendations for the best practitioners in the area.

This directory is not complete, because every practitioner listed must be a member of the National Center for Homeopathy and must pay a small fee for the listing, and many good practitioners do not need or want additional publicity. The directory is free to members of the National Center for Homeopathy. A free listing of homeopaths in your state is also available from Homeopathic Educational Services with any book order (www.homeopathic.com). For further recommendations of practitioners, consider checking out the following:

- *Your friends.* Asking your friends for recommendations is a tried-and-true way to find a homeopath. It is amazing how many people assume that their friends aren't into "this homeopathic stuff," but once the subject is broached discover that they and their family have been using these medicines for a long time and that they may be aware of a good homeopath in the area.
- *Health food stores.* Go to your local health food

stores and ask people who work in the homeopathic section for their recommendations.
Some people are more knowledgeable than
others, so you may have to check out a few
stores.

- *Homeopathic pharmacies.* Some pharmacies have
begun to specialize in homeopathy. Such
pharmacies are a great source for finding a
homeopath.
- *Conventional pharmacies that sell homeopathic medicines.*
A growing number of conventional pharmacies
sell a small number of homeopathic medicines.
However, only a small percentage of these
pharmacists will be adequately familiar with
local homeopaths.
- *Homeopathic study groups.* There are now several
hundred homeopathic study groups throughout
the United States. These are groups of people
(mostly women) with a special interest in
homeopathy. Because of this special interest,
they are usually knowledgeable about the best
homeopaths in their area. Contact the National
Center for Homeopathy or Homeopathic
Educational Services for a name and number of
a homeopathic study group closest to you.
- *Health and medical professionals.* Health and medical
professionals, especially those who use some
natural therapies themselves, are sometimes
familiar with local homeopaths.
- *Alternative newspapers and magazines.* Newspapers

and magazines that cover natural health and healing often have listings and advertisements for homeopaths.

- *The Yellow Pages.* You may be able to find homeopaths by simply looking in your Yellow Pages. However, because many homeopaths do not know that they can use this listing, the number of homeopaths in the book is usually limited.
- *The Internet.* There are now various alternative medicine forums on the Web with people discussing homeopathic and natural medicine. The Internet is a great place to find what you need.

more about finding the right homeopath

But how, you may be asking, do I know if a homeopath is any good? This question is actually more difficult to answer than it may seem. Although it is relatively easy to compare computer repair services, it is not as easy to compare homeopaths or other types of healers. Still, various specialty board certifications in homeopathy can give you the confidence that a practitioner with one of these degrees has a significant amount of knowledge about homeopathy:

- The "DHt." (a diplomat in homeotherapeutics) is available only to medical doctors (M.D.) and to osteopathic physicians (D.O.) from the American Board of Homeotherapeutics.

- The "DHANP" (Diplomat in the Homeopathic Academy of Naturopathic Physicians) certification is available only to naturopathic physicians (N.D.) who have graduated from accredited schools of naturopathic medicine and who are licensed in at least one state in the United States. (Be wary of naturopaths who have graduated from one of the mail-order naturopathic schools; this concern is not based on their knowledge or lack of it but on the fact that their training in homeopathy is inadequate for people wanting to be primary-care providers. Also, while distance learning education can be a great way to learn, many people, myself included, feel uncomfortable with the granting of "doctoral" degrees through mail order.)
- The "CCH" (Certification in Classical Homeopathy) is awarded to anyone who passes a rigorous examination given by the Council for Homeopathic Certification. Despite the fact that one doesn't have to be licensed in a conventional health profession to obtain this certification, the test for this degree is considered one of the most challenging by any homeopathic certifying agency. The certification does not guarantee the legal right to practice homeopathy, though it does convey to the public that the holder is knowledgeable of classical homeopathy.
- The "RSHom" refers to those who are

"Registered in the Society of Homeopaths." The Society of Homeopaths is an organization of professional homeopaths. Originally, it comprised only unlicensed practitioners, but now anyone can be a member, and its examination is the same as that developed by the Council for Homeopathic Certification.

Please note that because certification is not presently required to engage in homeopathic practice, many homeopaths have not sought to be certified. However, there are some general guidelines that can help a consumer determine if a homeopath is good. You are more likely to know that the practitioner is a high-quality homeopath if he or she:

- specializes in homeopathy as the primary treatment;
- prescribes constitutional medicines, not just remedies for acute or recurrent symptoms;
- asks you to describe each of your symptoms in great detail;
- conducts a first interview that lasts at least one hour;
- devotes a significant part of the interview to asking a series of detailed questions about your psychological state;
- uses a computer to help find the correct medicine;
- uses a book called a repertory in your presence (this may not be necessary if he or she has a computer).

People sometimes need to travel a few hundred or more miles to see a good homeopath. Despite the inconvenience, the special health benefits from quality homeopathic care make these efforts worth the extra cost and aggravation of traveling.

when to consider changing homeopaths

It is best to stay with one homeopath for many years. In fact, it is also best if other members of your family go to the same homeopath, because the homeopath is then able to understand you better and is usually more able to prescribe accurately when he or she sees people with your genetic heritage. The better your practitioner knows you, the more able he or she will be to find the correct remedies for you, both for acute and for chronic ailments.

It should be also acknowledged that some practitioners are unable to understand and effectively treat certain people. Also, a homeopath may be initially effective but then be unable to take the healing process to deeper levels. And at times, a homeopath may get into a rut in prescribing for a person and fail to prescribe some other remedies that should also be considered.

If your practitioner has not adequately helped to improve your health after a year, you may want to check in with him or her before changing practitioners. One option to consider is to ask that he or she consult with a colleague about your case. Another option is to ask your practitioner if it makes sense for you to actually see another homeopath. Complex or difficult cases can require that this new homeopath see you and conduct an in-depth interview. Your homeopath can be helpful in suggesting a colleague.

You should not consider changing homeopaths unless there has been no progress in your health for at least twelve months. It may be worthwhile to talk with your homeopath before changing practitioners, even though it may be difficult to be candid about your misgivings. There is actually a chance that the homeopath may help you acknowledge that there has been some progress in your health. Some people have a tendency to forget about the symptoms they once had when they are no longer experiencing them. A conversation with your practitioner may give you insight into yourself by helping you determine whether or not you have been in denial about your progress or if you have been too impatient in seeking significant changes in a limited time. On the other hand, this conversation may further confirm your desire to move on.

Because there is always the chance that you will return to your initial practitioner at some point, it is best to be up-front with him. Your change to another practitioner will inevitably come to his attention anyway, because you may want to have your files sent to the new practitioner so that she can benefit from knowing which remedies have or haven't worked for you.

If it is clear that you have experienced no progress in your health, and you feel that the homeopath does not adequately understand you and your symptoms, it may not be appropriate to seek another homeopath or a different type of homeopathic care. For uncertain reasons some people have conditions that do not seem to be easily treated with classical homeopathy. They may need a rare medicine that can more easily be discovered by a person practicing a more unconventional approach to homeopathy.

Since good healers recognize that there is no single way to heal people, they usually have an open mind to other methods, especially when theirs has not been effective.

the cost of professional homeopathic care

The cost of homeopathic care varies from one homeopath to another, from one city to another, and from one area to another. Medical doctors who practice homeopathy generally charge more than non-M.D.s, and the longer the practitioner has been in practice, the higher the fees tend to be. Homeopaths in large cities also tend to charge more than those in small cities or rural areas. And those homeopaths who teach other homeopaths tend to charge more than those who don't.

The first visit to a homeopath tends to last from sixty to ninety minutes. The fees of a homeopath with an M.D. will tend to be comparable with other physician specialists, ranging from $125.00 to $450.00. Other homeopaths charge from $50.00 to $250.00. Follow-up visits last between fifteen and forty-five minutes. M.D.s charge from $50.00 to $100.00, while non-M.D.s charge from $30.00 to $80.00.

Even though fees for care from homeopathic M.D.s tend to be similar to conventional physicians', the amount of time that homeopaths spend with their patients tends to be significantly longer. Homeopathic physicians earn good incomes, though they are generally not as high as the average medical doctor.

The cost of the homeopathic medicine is negligible. When only one medicine is prescribed (as is most common), it costs between $5.00 and $15.00. Some homeopaths do not charge for medicine.

The costs of homeopathic care, like the costs of all medical care, are high, but the costs of illness, especially chronic illness, are even higher. Some people may be tempted to treat themselves and to avoid professional homeopaths, but this decision can be more costly in the long run because it is not easy to treat chronic ailments with homeopathic medicine, unless one is very well trained in this system.

It should also be noted that homeopaths generally discourage frequent visits unless they are medically necessary, and that the time between visits ranges from one to six months. Because of this, the yearly cost of homeopathic care is considerably less than that of conventional medical care as well as of most types of alternative medicine. These factors do not even take into account the further cost savings that result from the ability of homeopathic medicines to strengthen one's immune system and prevent future costly diseases.

Also, medically trained homeopaths will recommend laboratory analysis when indicated, but they rarely need to run such tests to determine the appropriate homeopathic medicine. As a result, homeopaths tend to perform laboratory tests significantly less frequently than do conventional physicians, which further reduces healthcare costs. And the absence of side effects from homeopathic medicines further reduces the cost of care, since side effects usually lead to the need for more medical treatment.

On two separate occasions, the French government conducted cost-effectiveness studies on homeopathic medicine. They investigated the costs of treatment from a homeopathic physician and those of a conventional physician and discovered that homeopathic care costs were considerably cheaper. (Caisse Nationale de l'Assurance Maladie des Travailleurs Salariés, 1996 study of 130,000 prescriptions; [National Inter-Regulations System] 61, French Government Report, January 1991.)

insurance and homeopathy

Most insurance companies cover the care that most homeopaths provide, because the vast majority of professional homeopaths in the United States are licensed professionals such as medical doctors, osteopaths, chiropractors, acupuncturists, and naturopaths. Consumers must review their insurance to determine if they have

coverage from chiropractors, acupuncturists, and naturopaths. Although many insurers cover their care these
days, some policies allow only a limited number of visits. If your policy doesn't cover the care you want, instead
of changing insurance companies, consider contacting
the company or your insurance broker and informing
them of your interests. Only when consumers make their
desires heard will the insurance market change. Some
insurance companies actually specialize in coverage of
alternative health care. Look for their advertisements in
health magazines, or consult an insurance broker.

Insurance companies will rarely cover homeopathic
care by unlicensed professionals, though some policies
will cover their care when it is provided in a medical doctor's office and this doctor supervises the patient's care.

Insurance companies will not cover the small
expenses of homeopathic medicines, because they tend
to pay for prescription drugs only, and homeopathic
remedies are primarily over-the-counter drugs. Homeopathic medicines only cost $5 to $15 each, and because
they are over-the-counter drugs that do not require a
physician's prescription for purchase, insurance companies do not cover their cost.

treating yourself

Although any serious and/or chronic ailment requires the care of a professional homeopath, as discussed in the last chapter, you can learn to treat yourself and your family members for many common ailments. Because homeopathic medicines are so much safer than conventional ones (that is, there are no side effects and they do not suppress symptoms), people should consider using these safer medicines first and then resorting to riskier methods only when necessary.

You can learn to treat headaches, allergies, sinusitis, influenzas, sore throats, respiratory infections, teething, colic, ear infections, indigestion, bladder infections, P.M.S., vaginitis, arthritis, sprains and strains, cuts, burns, head injuries, and many other conditions. There are, however, certain extreme cases of any of these conditions that may constitute a medical emergency for which medical care, not self-care, should be sought.

The trick to getting the best results with homeopathic medicines is to individualize a remedy to your unique pattern of symptoms. In addition to using this book, I recommend that you consult other homeopathic guidebooks, and for those people who want to become particularly skilled in using homeopathic medicines, I recommend getting software that helps you to find the correct homeopathic medicine.

doses and potency

Generally, it is best to use the 6th, 12th, or 30th potency (written 6X, 6C, 12X, 12C, 30X, or 30C). The more confident you are that you are using the correct remedy, the higher potency you should use. Once you become more knowledgeable of homeopathic medicine, you can consider using higher potencies, including the 200th and 1,000th (written 1M, since M in Roman numerals is 1,000).

How often you take a homeopathic medicine depends on your condition and its intensity. The more intense the symptoms, the more necessary it is to repeat a remedy. During intense pain or discomfort, consider taking it every thirty minutes or every two hours. During mild pain or discomfort, consider taking it every four hours or just three times a day. Stop taking the remedy if:

- pain or discomfort is significantly reduced;
- no improvement is observed after forty-eight hours;
- symptoms disappear and reappear repeatedly. In that case, it is recommended that you seek professional homeopathic care for a deeper-acting homeopathic medicine;
- new symptoms develop that are particularly discomforting;
- any medical emergency occurs.

Homeopathic medicines stimulate and augment the body's own healing. These medicines are not vitamins that need to be taken daily; rather, they should be taken only when they are needed, like any other medicine. The basic idea is to take as few doses as necessary but as many doses as are needed.

paying attention to symptoms

When selecting a homeopathic medicine, pay attention to your symptoms, especially when:

- they are intense (that is, they stop you from engaging in your normal activities)
- they are unique
- they affect your whole person (that is, all of

you is cold instead of just your hands or feet)
- they are emotional or mental

I should note here that homeopaths use a broader definition of the term symptom. Homeopaths define a symptom as:

- anything that limits or reduces your freedom
- anything that reduces or increases any pain or discomfort (this is called a "modality")
- any change from what you normally experience

---

homeopathic remedies and conventional medicine

Many people have asked me whether it is possible to take conventional medicines and homeopathic remedies at the same time. The answer is yes, though homeopathic medicines often work rapidly and effectively enough that you do not always need to take conventional drugs. Conventional drugs work primarily on the physical level, while homeopathic medicines work on the energy and systemic levels. Because these two different kinds of medicines are working on different levels, they are not necessarily incompatible.

However, some conventional medicines are so strong that they suppress the immune system, thereby inhibiting the positive action of the homeopathic medicine. In such situations the individual must decide if he or she wishes to use the conventional or homeopathic medicine. Conventional drugs also tend to suppress or mask

a person's symptoms, sometimes making it more difficult to find the correct homeopathic medicine.

can anything neutralize the effects
of homeopathic medicines?

While homeopathic medicines and conventional medicines are not always incompatible, many people believe
that other things can neutralize the effects of homeopathic remedies. This is actually a complex and contro-
versial subject, because while some patients have had the
positive benefits of a homeopathic medicine neutralized
by certain substances or actions, the majority of people
do not experience such problems. For instance, some
people have found that drinking coffee, applying camphor (Tiger Balm) or mentholated products (such as
Bengay), or experiencing certain dental procedures
(tooth drilling) can neutralize the action of a remedy.

Such problems, however, tend to be the exception
rather than the rule. Since homeopathy is so popular
throughout Europe, it is hard to imagine that coffee is a
serious problem, considering how popular it is in those
countries. Also, for every instance when it has been
thought that camphor, menthol, and tooth drilling neutralize a homeopathic medicine, there are many more
instances when they haven't.

Despite this controversy, it does make sense to avoid
these potential problems during the first two weeks (or
so) after seeing a professional homeopath. Homeopaths

often simply prescribe one dose of one high-potency remedy, and these more powerful remedies tend to be more susceptible to being neutralized than lower-potency medicines. Because a visit to a homeopath commonly lasts for one to two hours and usually isn't cheap, it is best to do everything possible to reduce factors that may neutralize a remedy's action.

To properly care for your remedies so that they retain their potency, it is always best to store homeopathic medicines or a homeopathic medicine kit away from strong odors, direct light, or excessive heat. It is also best to keep a homeopathic medicine in its original container and not transfer it to another container, unless this new one has been sterilized.

homeopathic remedies

The first thing to keep in mind when considering treating yourself or a family member is that there is no one homeopathic for everyone with a specific disease or complaint. Usually, a homeopathic medicine must be individualized to the person and his or her unique pattern of symptoms. In this chapter I will describe some common complaints and then will list some of the remedies that are often indicated. However, you may need to consult other, more detailed homeopathic guidebooks to improve your accuracy when prescribing.

William Osler, M.D., considered the father of modern medicine, once said, "It is more important to know what type of person has a disease than it is to know what disease a person has." This wise statement is the premise on which homeopathy operates. As you will see when you read about the different homeopathic medicines, a remedy is not simply prescribed for a specific disease, but for the way the patient manifests it and for the type of person (mentally and emotionally) that he or she is.

And although some homeopathic medicines are known poisons, don't fret: homeopaths use such small doses of these substances that even the F.D.A. recognizes these remedies as safe. To determine the best dose and potency to use, please see chapter 6.

pregnancy and labor

Pregnancy and labor are great times to use homeopathic medicines, because they benefit both the mother and the fetus. Also, homeopathic medicines are considerably safer than conventional drugs. That said, pregnant or laboring women should see a professional homeopath for any chronic or serious ailment, though self-care is possible for many minor complaints.

One of the most common homeopathic medicines given to women in labor is *Arnica* (mountain daisy). It is a great remedy for the shock and trauma of labor, and it has a history of reducing bleeding. It should be taken internally in the 6th and 30th potency every other hour once labor has started, and *Arnica* ointment, gel, or spray

should be applied externally to the woman's back and pelvis to reduce the muscle aches of labor.

Morning Sickness

Sepia (the cuttlefish) is a common remedy for women who get morning sickness that is aggravated by simple motion or effort or who do not experience relief from not eating but are quickly relieved by eating crackers. Usually, women who need *Sepia* tend to get chilly easily and to be very irritable.

Pulsatilla (windflower) is indicated for emotional, moody, and weepy women who experience morning sickness. These women tend to be aggravated in a warm room and relieved in the open air.

Ipecacuanha (ipecac) is the remedy for women who suffer from severe and constant nausea that may even require hospitalization. Women who respond to *Ipecacuanha* also tend to experience profuse salivation.

---

treating infants

Children respond extremely well and rapidly to homeo-pathic medicines. What is even better news is that they love to take homeopathic medicines, since the remedies are usu-ally made with lactose or sucrose and thus tend to be sweet.

One of the most common remedies for infants is *Chamomilla* (chamomile), the best remedy for certain kinds of infants who are teething or who have colic, indi-gestion, or ear infections. *Chamomilla* is indicated when infants are extremely irritable. These infants throw tantrums, ask for things and then refuse them, and cry until they are held or carried. Typically, when *Chamomilla* is the correct remedy, the infant's health will improve within minutes. This remedy convinces many parents of the power of homeopathic medicines.

Another common homeopathic medicine for children is *Pulsatilla*, which is also indicated for certain kinds of infants who are teething or who have colic, indigestion, or ear infections. Infants who respond to *Pulsatilla* are very affectionate, desire attention, and crave sympathy. Although these infants cry, their crying is not sobbing, like the type of crying experienced by infants who respond to *Chamomilla*, but a sweet weeping that beckons the parent to hold and hug them. These infants tend to throw off their clothes and blanket and prefer being in the open or cool air (or at least have an open window).

Magnesia phosphorica (magnesium phosphate) is a good remedy for colic and sometimes for teething. It is indicated when infants experience cramping or pain in the abdomen that forces them to bend over. These infants are also relieved by warm applications on the abdomen or by warm drinks.

Diaper Rash

Calendula (marigold) is applied externally in ointment, gel, or spray form. *Calendula* is a very soothing and nutrient-rich herb that both reduces inflammation and heals the skin. *Calendula* is also available in soap form. It makes a wonderfully rich soap that is great for an infant's skin (and for those who want their skin to be as soft as an infant's).

Infants who experience recurrent diaper rashes and who do not adequately benefit from *Calendula* are recommended to seek professional homeopathic care for an individualized constitutional remedy.

Ear Infections

A recent study in a leading pediatric journal showed that individually chosen homeopathic medicines reduced ear infection symptoms in children as reported by their parents within the first twenty-four hours after treatment as compared to children who were given a placebo (Jacobs, Springer, and Crothers 2001).

Homeopathy is developing the reputation as the best treatment for this common pediatric complaint. *Chamomilla* and *Pulsatilla* are two important remedies to consider (for details about these two remedies, read the section above). Another important remedy for children with earaches is *Belladonna* (deadly nightshade). This remedy is indicated when the child has a reddened ear, ear canal, and eardrum, and even a flushed face. The pains are severe, throbbing, piercing, and may extend to the throat. The child may become agitated and in extreme cases may bite and/or scream. Sitting semierect and receiving warm applications provide temporary relief.

Mercurius (mercury) is a leading homeopathic medicine for ear infections accompanied by an offensive-smelling discharge. The pains may extend to the throat, and the child may have swollen glands and bad breath. Both hot and cold applications aggravate these children, and they tend to have such excessive salivation that they will wet their pillows with it.

the common cold

Homeopathy doesn't provide a cure for the common cold, but it does provide a cure for *people* with a common cold. This isn't simply a semantic issue. What I mean by that statement is that there is no single remedy that will cure everyone with a cold, but there are homeopathic remedies, when individually prescribed, that can and will cure a person with a cold.

Aconitum (monkshood) is called a "homeopathic vitamin C" and is a good remedy for the very first stages of a cold, especially if it started after exposure to cold air or wind. The person tends to have an increased thirst, a dry mouth, and perhaps a dry cough, and may begin to feel restless.

Allium cepa (onion) is a leading remedy for a person with a typical cold and who has a clear, watery nasal discharge that may burn and irritate the nostrils. Generally, the nasal discharge is worse in warm rooms and alleviated in the open air.

Pulsatilla is a remedy for children with an acute or chronic cold and who have a yellow or greenish nasal discharge that is worse at night and in warm rooms. Despite having a dry mouth, such children tend to be without thirst. This remedy is most commonly indicated with children who are sensitive, easily hurt, and crave attention and sympathy.

Arsenicum (arsenic) is a remedy for people who get chilled very easily and who experience a burning nasal discharge. These people tend to be thirsty but prefer only sips of water at a time.

Kali bichromicum (potassium bichromate) is a remedy for people with a stringy nasal discharge that is usually yellow. This is the type of cold that may later become sinusitis.

If you can't figure out which remedy to give or if the remedy you want isn't immediately available, you may want to try one of the many homeopathic combination remedies for the common cold that are available at most health food stores and pharmacies.

influenza

Several studies have confirmed the success in using homeopathic medicines to treat the flu. Despite conventional medicine's technological wonders, it does nothing for this common viral condition.

Oscillococcinum (duck liver and heart) is the best remedy for the flu, as long as you use it within the first forty-eight hours of the onset of symptoms. Three studies by three groups of independent researchers have consistently found that *Oscillococcinum* is effective in treating the flu and flulike symptoms (Papp, Schuback, Beck et al. 1998; Ferley et al. 1989). If you do not or cannot treat within the first forty-eight hours or if any of the remedies below describe the symptoms of the sick person, consider the following remedies:

Gelsemium (yellow jessamine) is a remedy for people with the flu who feel exhausted. These people have difficulty getting out of bed. Their arms and legs, in particular, feel tired, and their eyes droop. They may experience a headache in the back of their head, and they usually are not very thirsty.

Bryonia (wild hops) is indicated when people have musculoskeletal pains that are exacerbated by any type of motion. These people hate warm rooms and prefer to have cool air around them. They have a dry mouth and a great thirst. They may have a headache in the back of the head, and they tend to be very irritable and want to be left alone.

Eupatorium perfoliatum (boneset) is a remedy for people with the flu who experience pain in their bones. They may also experience chills, especially in the morning.

injuries

Conventional medicine may offer painkillers to those people with injuries, but while these drugs provide relief, they don't stimulate healing and some, in fact, tend to slow it down. In contrast, homeopathic medicines can help encourage the healing process after an injury.

Using homeopathic medicines to treat injuries is actually easier than using it for treating diseases. We all need a similar process to heal a cut, sprain, or fracture, and thus, there are specific remedies to help heal specific types of injuries. In comparison, when two people have a headache, they each need an individualized remedy to help them to heal their unique conditions.

Some formal research has shown that homeopathic medicines are effective in treating sprains and strains (Zell 1988) as well as the chronic symptoms of people suffering from head injury (Chapman, Weintraub, Milburn et al. 1999). (Please note that this study on the treatment of chronic symptoms from head injuries tested the use of individually chosen homeopathic medicines; homeopaths generally assume that chronic symptoms from head injury require this individualized care.)

Shock

Any course in first aid emphasizes the importance of treating a person who has been seriously injured for shock first. One should first apply conventional procedures, which include stopping any significant bleeding, having the person lie down, keeping his or her feet raised slightly, and making certain that the person is neither too hot nor too cold. Then, when possible and once permission is granted, give the person *Arnica* (mountain daisy). If the person is not only in shock but also feels terrorized, the most effective remedy is *Aconitum* (monkshood).

Sprains and Strains

The first homeopathic medicine to use for sprains or strains is *Arnica* (mountain daisy), which should be taken internally in the 6th or 30th potency and should be applied externally in an ointment, gel, or spray form. This remedy should be used during the first twelve to twenty-four hours after a sprain. After this, *Rhus toxico-dendron* (poison ivy) is the best remedy, especially if the injury pain is worse upon initial motion and is reduced as the person limbers up. If the injured area is sensitive to the touch or if it feels lame (that is, if it's extremely difficult to use without pain), use *Ruta* (rue).

Besides using any of the above individual medicines, you can also consider administering a mixture of homeopathic medicines specifically formulated for injuries. There are both internal and external applications for injuries. One formal study on the treatment of sprains and strains using a mixture of homeopathic medicines in an external application found statistically significant results (Zell 1988).

Fractures

It is of course recommended that you have a fracture or possible fracture X-rayed and then have the broken bone set in a cast or splint if necessary. Homeopathic medicines can be used to help allay the pain and to augment healing of the bones.

The most common remedy for fractures is *Symphytum* (comfrey). Another remedy is *Ruta* (rue), especially when a joint is fractured. Don't forget to also use *Arnica* (mountain daisy) immediately after fracture to help reduce the shock from the injury.

Cuts and Wounds

External applications of *Calendula* (marigold) are so effective in closing up cuts and wounds that it is not recommended for deep cuts or wounds, because it closes up the outer part of them too rapidly. *Calendula* is rich in carotenoids that help to nourish the skin and even has small amounts of salicylic acid (the active ingredient in aspirin) that helps to reduce the pain from the wound.

An external application of *Hypericum* (St. John's wort) is recommended for deep cuts.

insect bites and stings

Ledum (wild rosemary) is a great remedy for bites and stings when the pain is relieved by ice or cold applications. If there is much swelling and burning or stinging pain, consider using *Apis* (crushed bee). Some external applications of homeopathic formulas are also helpful in reducing the pain, itching, and discomfort from bites or stings. Some research has found them to be particularly effective (Hill, Stam, and van Haselen 1996).

allergies

Conventional medicine's approach to treating allergies is actually based on the basic homeopathic principle of treating "likes with like." Conventional allergists use small doses of whatever the person is allergic to. However, homeopaths use much smaller doses, and they often will individualize a remedy not simply to what the person is allergic to but to whatever substance will cause symptoms that are most similar to what the person is experiencing.

It should be noted that there is presently more

positive research on the homeopathic treatment of people with allergies than there is for any other condition (Taylor, Reilly, Llewellyn-Jones et al. 2000).

There are three basic strategies in homeopathy for treating someone with allergies. The most simple is to take one of the homeopathic combination remedies for allergies commonly available at pharmacies and health food stores. These remedies will usually include many common substances to which people are allergic, as well as other substances that cause allergy-like symptoms. The most common allergen is house dust mites. A homeopathic dose of this allergen is often very useful for people with respiratory allergies. Because this remedy is sometimes difficult to find, contact Homeopathic Educational Ser-vices or select homeopathic pharmacies if you can't find it.

The second approach is to find an individualized remedy for the acute stage of the allergy (such remedies will be described below). Both the first and the second approaches will provide benefit for the acute symptoms of the allergy but will not cure the person of allergies.

The third approach is to go to a professional homeopath for a "constitutional remedy," that is, one that is individually chosen for the person based on his or her genetics, health history, and the totality of physical and psychological symptoms presently experienced. A constitutional remedy has the potential of significantly reducing the frequency and intensity of a person's allergy symptoms and may even provide a cure for them.

Some of the common remedies for the above-described second approach include the following remedies:

Allium cepa (onion) is for people with allergies who have a running nose and watery eyes, with the discharge from the nose irritating the nostrils, while the moisture in their tears is bland and nonirritating. These symptoms worsen in a warm room or in heat and are alleviated in a cool room or environment or from being outside.

Euphrasia (eyebright) is good for people with a runny nose and watery eyes. However, unlike those for whom *Allium cepa* works as a remedy, these people have tears that irritate their eyelids and cheeks and have a runny nose that is bland and nonirritating to the nostrils. These symptoms are worse in the open air, at night, and when lying down.

If both the nasal discharge and the tears are burning, consider *Arsenicum* (arsenic), especially if the symptoms are worse on the right side of the body. Usually, people who respond to *Arsenicum* are very chilly and thirsty but want only sips of water at a time.

Ambrosia (ragweed) is useful for people allergic to this herb, and *Solidago* (goldenrod) is useful for people allergic to goldenrod.

If you have a stringy nasal discharge, consider using *Kali bichromicum* (potassium bichromate).

asthma

Ideally, it is best for people with asthma to receive professional homeopathic care, but in a pinch, self-prescribed homeopathic remedies can be wonderfully helpful. One major study on the homeopathic treatment of asthma was published in *The Lancet*. The researchers prescribed whatever substance the person was most allergic to (house dust mites was the most common substance) (Reilly, Taylor, Beattie et al. 1994), and this study discovered very positive results.

There are, however, too many other remedies that could be of potential help to be described in this short book. Consider consulting one of the many homeopathic guidebooks listed in the resources at the end of this book.

arthritis

One study on the treatment of people with rheumatoid arthritis found that 82 percent of patients prescribed an individually chosen homeopathic medicine experienced some relief of symptoms, while only 21 percent of patients prescribed a placebo experienced a similar degree of relief (Gibson 1980).

Several homeopathic medicines can be self-prescribed in the treatment of arthritis. These treatments provide helpful temporary relief, but if you want more significant improvement, it is recommended that you seek professional homeopathic care.

One of the most common remedies for the acute phase of various types of arthritis is *Rhus toxicodendron* (poison ivy). It is indicated when a person's joint pains are made worse by initial motion and in cold or wet weather and are relieved by continued motion. Also, the person who needs this remedy tends to become quite stiff during rest times.

When any type of motion aggravates a person's joint pains, consider using *Bryonia* (wild hops). People who respond to *Bryonia* tend to get relief when direct pressure is placed on the painful area. These people also tend to have a dry mouth, great thirst, and a tendency toward constipation.

Apis (crushed bee) is useful if a person's joints become swollen and painful in warm weather and are relieved by cold applications.

Some external applications of mixtures of homeopathic medicines are also effective, and one study found that a homeopathic external formula was as effective as a conventional nonsteroidal anti-inflammatory drug in the treatment of osteoarthritis of the knee (van Haselen and Fisher 2000). Another study showed that a different formula, taken internally, was as effective as acetaminophen for this same ailment (Shealy, Thomlinson, Cox, and Borgmeyer 1998).

premenstrual syndrome

Many useful homeopathic medicines can reduce the physical and psychological symptoms that women feel before and during their menstruation. The following remedies should be considered:

Pulsatilla (windflower) is indicated when the woman becomes very emotional, moody, and weepy before her menses. Women who respond to this medicine experience an increased desire for attention, affection, and sympathy.

They tend to be averse to and feel worse in warm or stuffy rooms, desire open air, and are usually without thirst.

Women who need *Magnesia phosphorica* (magnesium phosphate) primarily experience physical symptoms, especially cramping that is relieved by application of warmth or hard pressure.

Colocynthis (bitter cucumber) is good for women who experience sharp cramping pains who are relieved primarily from bending over. Women who need this remedy tend to be very irritable.

Belladonna (deadly nightshade) is indicated when a woman experiences cramping pains that may come and go rapidly and that are aggravated by motion or simply by being jarred.

Lachesis (bushmaster) is useful when a woman wakes to cramps that tend to become worse from the slightest touch or pressure, even from clothing (such women usually wear loose clothing). As soon as the woman's flow begins, her pains vanish.

In addition to the above remedies, you can consider taking one of the homeopathic combination remedies for P.M.S. If, however, you want more significant and long-term relief, it is highly recommended that you seek professional homeopathic care.

indigestion

Self-application of homeopathic medicines can be effective in treating acute indigestion, although people with chronic indigestion should seek the care of a professional homeopath.

Indigestion refers to a wide variety of digestive complaints, including heartburn, abdominal bloating, gas, eructation (burping), nausea, and vomiting. Many people incorrectly assume that such symptoms are the result of nutritional problems. While this is certainly true some of the time, indigestion can also be the result of various disease processes that reduce the ability of a person to digest and assimilate their foods. Indigestion can also be influenced by strong emotions that are felt during or shortly after eating.

In addition, some people tend to think they are allergic to a specific food that is causing their indigestion. This scenario is certainly possible, and a simple way to evaluate if this is the case is to take that food out of your diet and to carefully monitor your symptoms. Some foods, like corn, soy, or wheat can be difficult to eliminate from the diet, because many processed foods include by-products of these foods in them.

Homeopathic medicines can help improve a person's digestive process in the short and long term. However, long-term improvement generally requires professional homeopathic care, while the following remedies tend to provide short-term relief.

Arsenicum (arsenic): This is a leading remedy for indigestion when there are burning pains in the stomach or rectum, a great thirst but for only sips at a time (usually of warm drinks), chilliness with an aggravation from exposure to cold, a general restlessness, great exhaustion, and anxiety about one's health. People who respond to this remedy experience an aggravation of their symptoms at midnight and afterward. These people tend to vomit soon after eating or drinking, especially cold things. *Arsenicum* is a leading remedy for indigestion from food poisoning.

Pulsatilla (windflower): Commonly given to children and women, this remedy is known to alleviate indigestion or heartburn after eating fatty foods (such as ice cream and fried food) or pork, a lack of thirst, an aversion to stuffy rooms, and a desire for open air. Typically, people who respond to this remedy are highly emotional and desire sympathy and attention.

Ipecacuanha (ipecac root): This is a leading remedy for nausea and vomiting, especially when the nausea is persistent, even after vomiting. Other characteristic symptoms include a lack of thirst, nausea from the simple smell of food, increased salivation, and an uncoated tongue.

Nux vomica (poison nut): Digestive problems that start after overeating; overconsumption of alcohol, coffee, or drugs (therapeutic or recreational); or mental stress are commonly relieved by this remedy. Heartburn, nausea, and gas are usually accompanied by increased irritability and usually a headache, all of which tend to be worse upon waking and after eating. This is the leading homeopathic remedy for people with hangovers.

Bryonia (white bryony): People who feel digestive discomfort after any type of motion do well with this remedy. People who need this remedy tend to be constipated and irritable; they desire being alone and have a great thirst for cold liquids. Typically, these people have a feeling of pressure in their stomach, as though there was a stone there, and they feel nauseous, dizzy, and faint upon sitting up or standing.

Lycopodium (club moss): This is a leading remedy for people who experience bloating, gas, and belching. People who need this medicine have an abdomen that is sensitive to any pressure, whether from a belt or elastic waistband. Typically, their symptoms are worse between 4:00 P.M. and 8:00 P.M. and at 2:00 A.M. People who benefit from this remedy tend to crave sweets and to feel full after eating only a small amount of food, though this doesn't always stop them from eating.

Sulphur (sulfur): People who get heartburn from overeating or from eating the wrong foods and who may also suffer from early-morning diarrhea often benefit from this remedy. Typically, these people tend to feel a generalized heat from their body that makes exposure to cool or cold air feel good and leads to an aggravation of symptoms from warmth or heat.

For all these remedies, take the 6th, 12th, or 30th potency every two hours for two or three doses during intense discomfort and three times a day during mild symptoms. If no obvious improvement occurs within twenty-four hours, consider another remedy. Consider seeking professional homeopathic care if symptoms are severe, persistent, or recurring.

psychological problems

Homeopaths cannot treat a person without also treating their emotional and mental states. Homeopathic remedies are prescribed based on their ability to treat the whole person. Even the founder of the famed Menninger Clinic, Dr. Charles Frederick Menninger, was a homeopathic doctor who found value in treating all types of patients with homeopathic medicines.

One of the most common homeopathic medicines for people who experience grief from the loss of a loved one or from the breakup of a relationship is *Ignatia* (St. Ignatius' bean). Although this remedy is given more often to women, it can be useful to men and children too. People who need *Ignatia* are known to hold in their emotions initially and then explode. They do not simply cry; they sob. Their sadness, including their held-in sadness, is manifested in a tendency toward frequent sighing.

When people experience anxiety before a performance, a presentation, a test, or a job interview, the most common remedy is *Gelsemium* (yellow jessamine). It is particularly useful when the person trembles, has diarrhea, or experiences a headache.

When a person experiences various physical symptoms related to anger, you should consider using *Staphysagria* (stavesacre). This remedy is particularly useful to people who have been physically or sexually abused or discriminated against.

use your computer

The vast majority of practicing homeopaths in the United States use sophisticated software and expert systems to help them find the best, most individualized homeopathic medicine. While the average conventional doctor uses software primarily for billing patients and insurance companies, homeopaths use it to provide better care for their patients.

There are also some simple homeopathic software programs available to consumers. For details about the newest software, see Homeopathic Educational Services (listed in the resources).

references

Bellavite, Paolo, and Andrea Signorini. 2002. *Homeopathy: A Frontier in Medical Science.* Berkeley, CA: North Atlantic.

Belon, P., J. Cumps, M. Ennis et al. 1999. "Inhibition of Human Basophil Degranulation by Successive Histamine Dilutions: Results of a European Multi-centre Trial." *Inflammation Research* 48 (Suppl 1): 17–18.

Belougne-Malfatti, E., O. Aguejouf, F. Doutremepuich et al. 1998. "Combination of Two Doses of Acetyl Salicylic Acid: Experimental Study of Arterial Thrombosis." *Thrombosis Research* 90: 215–21.

Chapman, E., R. Weintraub, M. Milburn et al. 1999. "Homeopathic Treatment of Mild Traumatic Brain Injury: A Randomized, Double-Blind,

Placebo-Controlled Trial." *Journal of Head Trauma Rehabilitation* 14, no. 6 (December): 521–42.

Coulter, Harris, M.D. *Divided Legacy: The Conflict Between Homeopathy and the American Medical Association.* Berkeley, CA: North Atlantic, 1975.

Ferley, J. P. et al. 1989. "A Controlled Evaluation of a Homeopathic Preparation in the Treatment of Influenza-like Syndromes." *British Journal of Clinical Pharmacology* 27 (March): 329–35.

Gibson, R. G., S. M. Gibson, A. D. MacNeill, et al. 1980. "Homeopathic Therapy in Rheumatoid Arthritis: Evaluation by Double-Blind Clinical Therapeutic Trial," *British Journal of Clinical Pharmacology.* 9:453–459.

Hill, N., C. Stam, and R. A. van Haselen. 1996. "The Efficacy of Prrrikweg Gel in the Treatment of Insect Bites: A Double-Blind, Placebo-Controlled Clinical Trial." *Pharmacy World and Science* 18, no. 1: 35–41.

Jacobs, J., D. A. Springer, and D. Crothers. 2001. "Homeopathic Treatment of Acute Otitis Media in Children: A Preliminary Randomized Placebo-Controlled Trial." *Pediatric Infectious Disease Journal* 20, no. 2 (February): 177–83.

Jonas, W., Y. Lin, and F. Tortella. 2001. "Neuroprotection from Glutamate Toxicity with Ultra-Low Dose Glutamate." *Neuropharmacology and Neurotoxicity* 12, no. 2 (February): 335–39.

Kleijnen, J., P. Knipschild, and G. ter Riet. 1991. "Clinical Trials of Homeopathy." *British Medical Journal* 302 (February): 316–23.

Linde, K., N. Clausius, G. Ramirez et al. 1997. "Are the

Clinical Effects of Homeopathy Placebo Effects? A Meta-Analysis of Placebo-Controlled Trials." *Lancet* 350 (September); 834–43.

Linde, K., W. B. Jonas, D. Melchart et al. 1994. "Critical Review and Meta-Analysis of Serial Agitated Dilutions in Experimental Toxicology." *Human and Experimental Toxicology* 13: 481–92.

Lo, S. Y. and B. Bonavida. 1988. "Physical, Chemical, and Biological Properties of Stable Water Clusters." Singapore: World Scientific.

Papp, R., G. Schuback, E. Beck et al. 1998. "Oscilloccinum in Patients with Influenza-like Syndromes: A Placebo-Controlled Double-Blind Evaluation." *British Homeopathic Journal* 87 (April): 69–76.

Reilly, David, Morag Taylor, Neil Beattie et al. 1994. "Is Evidence for Homeopathy Reproducible?" *Lancet* 344 (December): 1601–6.

Shealy, C. N., R. P. Thomlinson, R. H. Cox, and V. Borgmeyer. 1998. "Osteoarthritis Pain: A Comparison of Homeopathy and Acetaminophen." *American Journal of Pain Management* 8: 89–91.

Starr, Paul. 1982. The Social Transformation of American Medicine. New York: Basic.

Taylor, M. A., D. Reilly, R. H. Llewellyn-Jones et al. 2000. "Randomised Controlled Trial of Homeopathy versus Placebo in Perennial Allergic Rhinitis with Overview of Four Trial Series." *British Medical Journal* 321 (August): 471–76.

Ullman, Dana. 1995. *The Consumer's Guide to Homeopathy.* New York: Jeremy Tarcher/Putnam.

van Haselen, R. A., and P. A. Fisher. 2000. "A Randomized Controlled Trial Comparing Topical Piroxicam Gel with a Homeopathic Gel in Osteoarthritis of the Knee." *Rheumatology* 39 (2000): 714–19.

Zell, Jurgen, W. D. Connert, J. Mau et al. 1989. "Treatment of Acute Sprains of the Ankle: A Controlled Double-Blind Trial to Test the Effectiveness of a Homeopathic Ointment." *Biological Therapy* 7, no. 1: 1–6. Originally published in *Fortschritte der Medizin* 106, no. 5 (1988): 99–100.

homeopathy resources

This short body of information could not possibly include all the information that one needs to know about homeopathy. The following resources, however, provide valuable information for anyone who wants to know more about using homeopathic medicines for themselves and for their family as well as for anyone interested in pursuing a career in the field.

suggested reading

Introductory and Family Guidebooks
Bellavite, Paolo, and Andrea Signorini. 2002. *Homeopathy: A Frontier in Medical Science.* Berkeley, CA: North Atlantic.

Castro, Miranda. 1990. *The Complete Homeopathy Handbook.* New York: St. Martin's Press.

Cummings, Stephen, and Dana Ullman. 1997. *Everybody's Guide to Homeopathic Medicines.* New York: Jeremy Tarcher/Putnam.

Grossinger, Richard. 1998. *Homeopathy: The Great Riddle.* Berkeley, CA: North Atlantic.

Hershoff, Asa. 1999. *Homeopathic Remedies: A Rapid Guide.* New York: Avery.

Kruzel, Thomas. 1992. *Homeopathic Emergency Guide.* Berkeley, CA: North Atlantic.

Lockie, Andrew. 1993. *The Family Guide to Homeopathy.* New York: Fireside.

Panos, Maesimund, and Jane Heimlich. 1980. *Homeopathic Medicine at Home.* New York: Jeremy Tarcher.

Skinner, Sidney. 2001. *Homeopathic Medicines in Primary Care.* Gaithersburg, MD: Aspen.

Ullman, Dana. 1995. *The Consumer's Guide to Homeopathy.* New York: Jeremy Tarcher/Putnam.

————. 1991. *Discovering Homeopathy: Medicine for the 21st Century.* Berkeley, CA: North Atlantic.

————. 1999. *Homeopathy A–Z.* Carlsbad, CA: Hay House.

Vithoulkas, George. 1980. *The Science of Homeopathy.* New York: Grove.

Whitmont, Edward C. 1993. *The Alchemy of Healing.* Berkeley, CA: North Atlantic.

Specialized Self-Care Books

Bailey, Philip. 1995. *Homeopathic Psychology.* Berkeley, CA: North Atlantic.

Castro, Miranda. 1993. *Homeopathy for Pregnancy, Birth and Your Baby's First Year.* New York: St. Martin's Press.

Hamilton, Don. 1999. *Homeopathic Care for Cats and Dogs.* Berkeley, CA: North Atlantic.

Hershoff, Asa. 1996. *Homeopathy for Musculoskeletal Healing.* Berkeley, CA: North Atlantic.

Lockie, Andrew, and Nicola Geddes. 1994. *The Women's Guide to Homeopathy.* New York: St. Martin's Press.

Moskowitz, Richard. 1992. *Homeopathic Medicine for Pregnancy and Childbirth.* Berkeley, CA: North Atlantic.

Reichenberg-Ullman, Judyth. 2000. *Whole Woman Homeopathy.* Rocklin, CA: Prima.

Reichenberg-Ullman, Judyth and Robert Ullman. 2002. *Prozac Free.* Berkeley, CA: North Atlantic.

————. 1998. *The Quick and Simple Guide to Homeopathic Self-Care.* Rocklin, CA: Prima.

————. 1998. *Rage-Free Kids.* Rocklin, CA: Prima.

————. 1996. *Ritalin-Free Kids.* Rocklin, CA: Prima.

Schmidt, Michael A. 1990. *Healing Childhood Ear Infections: Causes, Prevention, and Alternative Treatment.* Berkeley, CA: North Atlantic.

Souter, Keith. 1993. *Homeopathy for the Third Age.* Walden, Eng.: C. W. Daniel.

Subotnick, Steven. 1991. *Sports and Exercise Injuries: Conventional, Homeopathic, and Alternative Treatments.* Berkeley, CA: North Atlantic.

Ullman, Dana. 1992. *Homeopathic Medicine for Children and Infants.* New York: Jeremy Tarcher/Putnam.

————. 2000. *The One Minute (Or So) Healer: More Wisdom from the Sages, the Rosemarys, and the Times.* Carlsbad, CA: Hay House.

————. 1999. *The Steps to Healing: Wisdom from the Sages, the Rosemarys, and the Times.* Carlsbad, CA: Hay House.

Zand, Janet, Rachel Walton, and Bob Rountree. 1994. *Smart Medicine for a Healthier Child.* New York: Avery.

homeopathic internet sites

The following listing of sites dealing with homeopathic medicine is not meant to be complete. The sites listed below that also sell products (books, medicines, software, and so on) are listed only if the information they provide supercedes their emphasis on sales.

Homeopathy Home Page

www.homeopathyhome.com

This website provides links to various homeopathic resources and websites throughout the Internet. You can also subscribe, without cost, to a homeopathic discussion group or access various past discussion topics by searching their tables of content. You can also find links to commercial and noncommercial sites in homeopathy (and in various languages).

Homeopathic Educational Services

www.homeopathic.com

This site provides more than one hundred articles on homeopathic principles, self-care, professional care, clinical and laboratory research, and how to use homeopathic medicines for home care of various acute ailments. It also contains an extensive catalog of homeopathic books, tapes, medicines, software, and correspondence courses. They will send you a free list of homeopathic practitioners in your U.S. state upon request with any book order.

The National Center for Homeopathy
www.homeopathic.org

The N.C.H. is the leading homeopathic organization in the United States. This site includes several dozen articles plus a searchable directory of homeopaths in the United States. The site also contains up-to-date references to a large number of media reports on homeopathy and to various leading clinical and laboratory research studies.

Homeopathic Online Discussion Groups

There are two truly wonderful online discussion groups that focus primarily on homeopathy. One is called "lyghtforce," and believe it or not, there are from fifteen to fifty postings each day. You can subscribe to it in two ways, either with each individual posting or as one long "digest" (with an initial and invaluable table of contents). Go to www.lyghtforce.com. Also, some discussion takes place at www.homeopathyhome.com.

Hahnemann's Advanced Teachings (with David Little)
www.simillimum.com

This is a site for serious students of classical homeopathy. Developed by a master homeopath, David Little, this

site provides detailed instruction in Hahnemannian homeopathy. You can also subscribe to further online training.

Dr. Will Taylor's Site
www.simillibus.com

An M.D./homeopath developed this site, which
includes a lot of good information for serious students
and practitioners of homeopathy, with a primary focus
on classical homeopathy.

North American Society of Homeopaths (N.A.S.H.)
www.homeopathy.org

This is the leading organization of unlicensed professional homeopaths.

Homeopathic Directory
www.homeopathicdirectory.com

This site is an online directory to homeopaths who have
passed an examination given by one or more respected homeopathic certifying agencies. Although this is a very useful directory, only a small number of homeopaths have sought to be
certified. Because of this, this directory is limited.

---

source of homeopathic books, tapes, software, and distance-learning courses

---

Homeopathic Educational Services
www.homeopathic.com; mail@homeopathic.com

This is the leading resource for homeopathic
books, tapes, medicines, medicine kits, software, and

correspondence courses. You can also write them at 2124 Kittredge St., Berkeley, CA 94704, or call at (510) 649-0294.

homeopathic organizations

National Center for Homeopathy
801 N. Fairfax #306
Alexandria, VA 22314
(703) 548-7790
www.homeopathic.org

American Institute of Homeopathy
801 N. Fairfax #306
Alexandria, VA 22314
(703) 548-7790

homeopathic schools and training programs

American University of Complementary Medicine
11543 Olympic Blvd.
Los Angeles, CA 90064
(310) 914-4116
www.aucm.org

Bastyr University
14500 Juanita Dr. N.E.
Bothell, WA 98011
(425) 823-1300
www.bastyr.edu

British Institute of Homeopathy
(correspondence course also available through
Homeopathic Educational Services)
580 Zion Rd.
Egg Harbor, NJ 08234
(609) 927-7327
www.britinsthom.com

Caduceus Institute of Classical Homeopathy
516 Caledonia
Santa Cruz, CA 95012
(800) 396-9778 or (831) 466-0516
www.homeopathyhome.com/caduceus

Canadian Academy of Homeopathy
1173 boul. du Mont-Royal
Outremont, QC H2V 2H6
(514) 279-6629
www.homeopathy.ca

Canadian College of Naturopathic Medicine
1255 Sheppard Ave. E.
N. York, ON M2K 1E2
(416) 498-1255
www.ccnm.edu

Colorado Institute for Classical Homeopathy
2299 Pearl St. #400
Boulder, CO 80302
(303) 440-3717
www.coloradohomeopathyschool.org

Desert Institute School of Classical Homeopathy
2001 W. Camelback Rd. #150
Phoenix, AZ 85015
(602) 347-7950
www.chiaz.com

Evolution of the Self School of Homeopathy
2700 Woodlands Village #300-250
Flagstaff, AZ 86001
(520) 525-2228

Five Elements Center
P.O. Box 537
Boonton, NJ 07005
(973) 402-8510

Hahnemann Center for Homeopathy
and Heilkunst
1445 St. Joseph Blvd.
Ottawa, ON K1C 7K9
(613) 830-2556
www.homeopathy.com

Hahnemann Medical College
Lindsay Hall
235 Washington Ave.
Point Richmond, CA 94801
(510) 232-2079
www.hahnemanncollege.com

Homeopathic Academy of Southern California
2136 Oxford Ave.
Cardiff by the Sea, CA 92007
(858) 794-0787
www.homeopathic-academy.com

Hudson Valley School of Classical Homeopathy
321 McKinstry Rd.
Gardiner, NY 12525
(845) 255-6141
www.classicalhomeopathy.com

International Academy of Classical Homeopathy
P.O. Box 24
Gardiner, NY 12525
(845) 255-6141

Institute of Classical Homeopathy
1336-D Oak Ave.
St. Helena, CA 94574
(707) 963-7796
www.classicalhomeopathy.org

Luminos Homeopathic Courses
F-31 C. O. Bowen Island,
BC V0N 1G0
(604) 947-0757
www.homeopathycourses.com

Maui Academy of Homeopathy
P.O. Box 880400
Pukalani, HI 96788
(808) 572-2229
www.mauiacademy.com

National College of Naturopathic Medicine
049 S.W. Porter
Portland, OR 97201
(503) 499-4343
www.ncnm.edu

New England School of Homeopathy
356 Middle St.
Amherst, MA 01002
(413) 256-5949
www.nesh.com

Northwestern Academy of Homeopathy
10700 Old County Rd. #15
Minneapolis, MN 55441
(612) 794-6445
www.homeopathicschool.org

Pacific Academy of Homeopathy
1199 Sanchez St.
San Francisco, CA 94114
(415) 695-2710
www.homeopathy-academy.org

Professional Course in Veterinary Homeopathy
1283 Lincoln St.
Eugene, OR 97401
(541) 342-7665
www.drpitcairn.com

Renaissance Institute of Classical Homeopathy
P.O. Box 31025
Santa Fe, NM 87594
(505) 982-9273
www.drluc.com

School of Homeopahty, New York
964 Third Ave., Eighth Floor
New York, NY 10155
(212) 570-2576
www.homeopathyschool.com

Southwest College of Naturopathic Medicine
2140 E. Broadway Rd.
Tempe, AZ 85282
(480) 858-9100
www.scnm.edu

Teleosis School of Homeopathy
333 W. Fifty-sixth St. #1C
New York, NY 10019
(212) 977-8118
www.teleosis.com

Texas Institute for Homeopathy
876 Amberstone
San Antonio, TX 78258
(800) 460-7580
www.texashomeopathy.com

Toronto School of Homeopathic Medicine
17 Yorkville Ave. #200
Toronto, ON M4W ILI
(416) 966-2350
www.homeopathycanada.com

University of Bridgeport
College of Naturopathic Medicine
60 Lafayette Blvd.
Bridgeport, CT 06601
(800) 392-3582
www.bridgeport.edu/naturopathy/index.html

Vancouver Homeopathic Academy
P.O. Box 34095, Station D
Vancouver, BC V6J 4MI
(604) 708-9387

homeopathic certification organizations

Academy of Veterinary Homeopathy
6400 E. Independence Blvd.
Charlotte, NC 28212
(704) 535-6688
www.avh.org

American Board of Homeotherapeutics
617 W. Main St., Fourth floor
Charlottesville, VA 22903
(703) 548-7790

The Council for Homeopathic Certification
P.O. Box 12180
La Crescenta, CA 91224-0880
(866) 242-3399
www.homeopathicdirectory.com/old

Homeopathic Academy of Naturopathic Physicians
12132 S.E. Foster Place
Portland, OR 97226
(503) 761-3298
www.healthy.net/hanp

North American Society of Homeopaths
1122 Pike St.
Seattle, WA. 98122
(206) 720-7000
www.homeopathy.org

index

C

D

I

about the author

D ana Ullman has been involved in homeopathic medicine since 1972. He holds a master's degree in public health from the University of California at Berkeley. Mr. Ullman has consulted for the World Health Organization and teaches in various parts of the world. He serves as a member of the Advisory Council of the Alternative Medicine Center at Columbia University's College of Physicians and Surgeons, as consultant to Harvard Medical School's Center to Assess Alternative Therapy for Chronic Illness, and as an adjunct faculty member at the University of Arizona School of Medicine. Mr. Ullman is president of the Foundation for Homeopathic Education and Research, the director of Homeopathic Educational Services, and a publisher and distributor of homeopathic informational products and a resource center for homeopathic medicines.

Dana Ullman has formulated a line of homeopathic medcines for children, women, and families for Nature's Way, a leading manufacturer of natural medicines.

Mr. Ullman has written several books on homeopathy, including *Homeopathic Medicine for Children and Infants, Homeopathy A—Z,* and *The Consumer's Guide to Homeopathy.*

If you enjoyed *Essential Homeopathy*, we recommend the following books from New World Library/H J Kramer.

Aromatherapy for the Healthy Child by Valerie Ann Worwood. This is the definitive book on how to promote health, prevent illness, and treat minor ailments in children using safe and natural aromatherapy at home.

The Complete Book of Essential Oils & Aromatherapy by Valerie Ann Worwood. An encyclopedic book containing every conceivable use for essential oils and aromatherapy in everyday life.

Essential Aromatherapy by Susan Worwood. This book is lively A-to-Z reference on the preparation and use of essential oils as holistic healing agents.

The Fragrant Heavens by Valerie Ann Worwood. In this new volume, Valerie Ann Worwood — one of the world's leading authorities on aromatherapy — explores the connection between fragrance and spirituality.

The Fragrant Mind by Valerie Ann Worwood. This groundbreaking book paves a new way for the uses of aromatherapy, concentrating on the mood-changing effects of essential oils.

Guided Imagery for Self-Healing by Martin L. Rossman, M.D. Using methods he has taught to thousands of patients and health-care professionals since 1972, Dr.

Rossman teaches a step-by-step method of harnessing the power of the mind to further one's own physical healing.

Massage for Busy People by Dawn Groves. More than twenty-five demonstrative photographs in this easy-to-understand how-to text provide a description of the various types of self-massage techniques to de-stress and relax.

Meditation — The Complete Guide by Patricia Monaghan and Eleanor G. Viereck. This authoritative reference work provides a clear explanation of more than thirty-five meditation practices. Whether you are new to meditation or have had years of experience, you will find this to be an invaluable guide.

Meditation for Busy People by Dawn Groves. This concise, jargon-free guide introduces a simple method for fitting meditation into a complex and busy lifestyle.

Reclaiming Our Health by John Robbins. *Reclaiming our Health* is a provocative and crystal-clear commentary on one of the most complex issues facing America today — national health care.

Scents & Scentuality by Valerie Ann Worwood. By the world's leading aromatherapist, this is the essential guide to aromatherapy for helping you discover your true romantic self.

The Tao of Healing by Haven Treviño. In eighty-one inspiring meditations, the poetic wisdom of the Tao Te Ching is applied to healing as a natural art.

The Vegetarian Lunchbasket by Linda Haynes. The new edition of this popular cookbook contains more than 225 great recipes for breads, spreads, soups, sandwiches, condiments, main dishes, and desserts that are lowfat, tasty, and vegetarian.

Yoga for Busy People by Dawn Groves. Dawn Groves introduces the ancient art of yoga to the overworked bodies and stressed-out minds of busy people everywhere. Her down-to-earth, practical, and easy-to-follow method helps readers create a yoga routine that provides maximum value in minimum time.